From Intern To Attending

Dr. Alhad Naragude
Vishakha N Punjani

Peepee Publishers and Distributors Private Limited®

From Intern To Attending

Published by
Pawaninder P. Vij and Anupam Vij

Peepee Publishers and Distributors Private Limited
Head Office: 160, Shakti Vihar, Pitam Pura, Delhi-110 034 (India)

Correspondence Address:

7/31, First Floor, Ansari Road, Daryaganj
New Delhi-110 002 (India)

Ph: 41512412, 9811156083

e-mail: peepee160@yahoo.co.in

e-mail: peepee160@gmail.com

www.peepeepub.com

join us on facebook.com/pp.publishers

First Edition: 2025

ISBN: 978-81-9720-721-1

Foreword

Mark Twain said "We should be careful to get out of an experience only the wisdom that is in it and stop there; lest we be like the cat that sits down on a hot stove-lid. She will never sit down on a hot stove-lid again and that is well; but also she will never sit down on a cold one anymore."

Becoming a consultant is like running a marathon with a backpack full of medical textbooks—it's tough; it's long; and it's definitely not for the faint of heart. This journey demands more than just knowing your stuff; it's a full-on test of how much grit and determination you've got. It also requires a deep commitment to patient care—because saving lives is an important profession. As you transition from the bright-eyed, bushy-tailed medical student phase into the wild world of residency, you'll encounter a learning curve that feels more like a cliff. You'll be expected to take all that theory you've crammed into your brain and actually use it in real life. A good student learns the difference between life and death, but a great doctor knows that it's just as important to be a decent human being who can talk to people without scaring them.

That's where this manual comes in. Think of it as your survival guide—your trusty companion as you navigate the unpredictable waters of residency. It's packed with advice and insights from fellow young doctor who has already walked this path and lived to tell the tale. Whether you're trying to master the art of surgery, survive your time on the wards, or just figure out how to make it through another 24-hour shift without crying, this book has got your back.

Section A of the book tackles the million-dollar question: "How to Choose a Specialty and Residency Program?" Let's be honest—choosing a specialty is like being at a buffet with too many options, except instead of deciding between chicken or paneer, you're choosing your entire future. Do you go with a government program, a private institution, or maybe just flip a coin? And then there's the real brain-teaser: which branch of medicine do you dive into? It's a decision that makes choosing a Netflix show look like a breeze. Fortunately, this manual is here to help, offering simple examples to guide you through the decision-making maze without losing your mind. There's also a chapter dedicated on "How to Prepare for Residency?" It's the pep talk you didn't know you needed to gear up for the long haul of training, helping you face the years ahead with something resembling confidence—or at least less panic.

Section B of the book dives into some of the more challenging aspects of residency, like "What to Expect During Residency?" (*Hint:* Expect everything.) It also covers vital topics such as "Mental Health," "Physical Health," and "Nutrition"—because in a residency program that lasts three or four years, keeping your sanity and your body intact is kind of important. The tips in this book are designed to help you navigate these tricky areas so that you can survive the grind without completely losing your marbles.

Relationships are a big deal too, and the book doesn't skimp on advice in that department. It covers the ups, downs, and sideways of relationships in the life of a young doctor, giving them the attention they deserve. And let's not forget finances—because while we're taught how to save lives, nobody ever teaches us how to save our wallets. As Robert Kiyosaki wisely said, "Financial freedom is available to those who learn about it and work for it." And it's painfully true for doctors. The book includes a chapter that educates you on all the fun stuff-like financial planning, tax strategies, loans, and budgeting. There's even an online link to an expert on tax planning! Honestly, I wish I'd known half of this when I was slogging through my residency.

And finally, as the book so aptly puts it in the chapter on Exercise, Nutrition, and Health: "Stress, Sweat, and Self-Care—The Trifecta of Neglect," doctors at every level are experts at putting work first and their own well-being somewhere around 37th place. It's a solid reminder that while we're busy saving lives, we're often neglecting our own mental and physical health.

In these pages, you'll not only get the technical know-how but also some good old-fashioned wisdom on the softer skills that are just as crucial for your journey to becoming a consultant. Whether it's communication, teamwork, leadership, or making ethical decisions without breaking a sweat, this manual covers it all. The authors understand that being a doctor is as much about the art of healing as it is about the science, and they've packed this book with the tools you need to master both without losing your mind in the process. As you dive into this journey, remember that every challenge is just an opportunity in disguise. Those long hours, self-doubt, and the occasional setbacks are all just part of the grand adventure that will eventually mold you into a consultant who not only meets but exceeds the highest standards of excellence and compassion. This manual is your trusty sidekick, ready to offer guidance, support, and the occasional pep talk to remind you that you're not alone in this marathon.

May this book be your secret weapon during residency and beyond, helping you transform from a competent specialist into an exemplary one. I highly recommend sharing this gem with anyone in medical training—it's packed with vital pearls of wisdom from young doctors who've survived the same rollercoaster and lived to tell the tale.

Best of luck on your quest to becoming a super-duper, all-star specialist doctor! May your stethoscope be ever shiny and your coffee supply never run dry.

Dr. Subodh Shivde
MS, MCh, FRCS (UROL), FRCS (EDIN, GLASG), Fellow European Board of Urology, Diploma in Laparoscopic Urology

Senior Consultant
DrNB Trainer & Coordinator
Department of Urology, Transplant and Robotics
Deenanath Mangeshkar Hospital and Research Centre
Pune, Maharashtra
India

Preface

"From Intern to Attending" is more than just a guide—it's a companion for medical students embarking on the transformative journey of residency. Designed for those on the cusp of entering or already immersed in their residency, this book offers a thoughtful exploration of how to navigate this pivotal phase of medical training.

The journey begins with guidance on selecting the right specialty and residency program, ensuring that you start on a path aligned with your preferences and strengths. It delves into the heart of residency, tackling the multifaceted challenges that lie ahead—balancing mental health amidst stress, maintaining relationships under time constraints, managing finances in a demanding environment, and preserving physical health when self-care often takes a backseat.

Residency is not just a professional transition but a profound personal evolution. As you shift from student to a responsible attending consultant, entrusted with patients' lives, this book offers insights to help you navigate these responsibilities with confidence. Through practical advice and real-world scenarios especially in India, "From Intern to Attending" equips you to handle the pressures, embrace the growth, and emerge not just as a skilled doctor, but as a resilient and well-rounded individual ready to lead in the medical field.

Dr. Alhad Naragude & Vishakha N Punjani

About The Authors

Dr. Alhad Naragude

Dr. Alhad Naragude completed his MBBS from BJGMC, Pune, followed by MS General Surgery from LTMMC, Mumbai. He wrote his first book – "NEET SS: Review of General Surgery for NEET/INI SS" at the end of his residency. The book helped residents to review Sabiston's Textbook of Surgery and served as a useful aid to crack Neet SS. Dr. Alhad is currently pursuing Urology Residency at Deenanath Mangeshkar Hospital and Research Centre, Pune.

Vishakha N Punjani

Vishakha N. Punjani, a clinical psychologist and psychotherapist, is a co-founder of Astitva Mental Health Clinic in Matunga, Mumbai. She is a clinical psychologist at the Department of Psychiatry, OPD-21, Lokmanya Tilak Municipal Medical College & Hospital, Sion, Mumbai. Being a practitioner with a penchant for research, she has contributed as an assistant junior researcher at the Department of Evolutionary and Neurosciences, Oxford University, United Kingdom. Her passion for conducting mental health and wellbeing workshops and interacting with people has led her to expand her horizons by providing training and support to the Indian Army. Moreover, she is a consultant at the Pre-Litigation Centre, High Court of Bombay, and an executive committee member of the Maharashtra State Legal Services Authority, Government of Maharashtra.

Acknowledgements

A huge thanks to my parents, Mr. Ulhas Naragude and Mrs. Usha Naragude, for raising me with just the right balance of love and discipline. Their support shaped me into the person who now knows way too much about obscure medical conditions. Shoutout to my siblings, who bravely endured the grueling residency marathon before me. They gave me the playbook, warned me about the pitfalls, and reassured me that the dark circles under my eyes and the receding hairline were just part of the "doctor" look.

To my soon-to-be wife, Dr. Shalvi Kamat, who not only proofread countless drafts of this book but also politely nudged me to finish it. Without her, this book would be eternally stuck in chapter one. Big thanks to Dr. Kiran Wakade and Dr. Devesh Shilimkar, my unofficial editors who generously lent their time, perspective, and red pens to this project. Tanvi and Anaya Kamat for designing the wonderful coverpage from scratch.

And of course, my co-JRs and colleagues, without whom my residency experience would have been like a bad sitcom with no laugh track. You all made the sleepless nights and endless rounds bearable—and occasionally even fun. Lastly, to my mentors and the ever-patient hospital staff who, day after day, let me make mistakes, learn from them, and trusted me to be a doctor.

Dr. Alhad Naragude

I would like to express my deepest gratitude to my *dadu-dadi* and *nana-nani* for their timeless wisdom, endless love, and the stories that shaped my values. To my incredible parents, Nilesh and Archana Punjani, thank you for your constant support, guidance, and for believing in me even when I doubted myself. To my wonderfully silly yet ever-supportive brother, Jay N Punjani, thank you for being my partner in laughter, challenges, and everything in between. You've kept me grounded through the ups and downs, and you never let me take myself too seriously.

A special thank you goes to my mentor, Sir Manohar B Watharkar, whose guidance has been nothing short of extraordinary. You've shaped my path with wisdom and patience, challenging me to think bigger, learn more, and push myself to new heights. I am forever grateful to you for teaching me that we as humans are more than this existence, and it's okay to not be moving around with my why's always. Thank you, Sir.

To my joint-founder, Heta N Shah, thank you for being my sounding board, my collaborator, and unpaid therapist.

Finally, I want to extend my heartfelt appreciation to all my patients, students and medical residents I have had the privilege to work with – thank you for having your faith in me! Your dedication, compassion, and tireless work ethic are inspiring. You remind me every day of why we do what we do, and I am honored to be a part of your journey. Keep pushing boundaries, and know that your efforts are shaping the future of medicine.

Vishakha N Punjani

TABLE OF CONTENTS

INTRODUCTION

Welcome to the journey through Medical Residency. Whether you're just starting Medical School, just got into the residency of your choice, or you're already a full-fledged Resident (and perpetually overwhelmed), we have made an effort to compile all the answers you're looking for. The path to become a doctor can seem like a stressful and painfully confusing maze, but with this guide, you can prepare yourself for what to expect every step of the way.

The guide is broken down into few main sections:

A. What To Do before Residency?

1. How to choose a specialty?
2. How to choose a residency program?
3. Preparing for residency

B. What To Expect during Residency?

4. The residency
5. Mental health
6. Relationships
7. Physical health and nutrition
8. Finances

Section—A

What To Do before Residency?

1. **How to choose a specialty?**
2. **How to choose a residency program?**
3. **Preparing for residency**

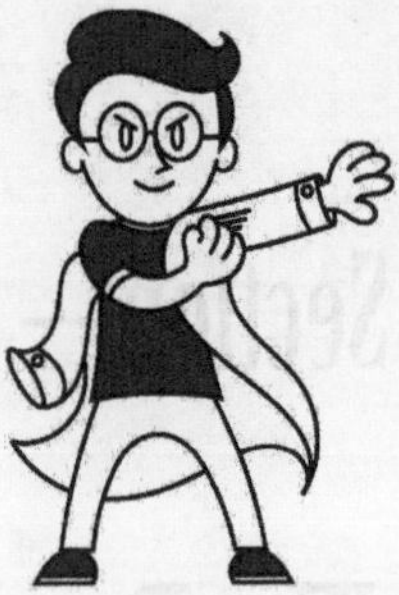

Got a rank in NEET PG?
Going through counselling?
Getting excited to become a part of a hospital team?

You're going to enter a phase of life which is transformative in all aspects of your overall development, not just as a doctor but as a person as well.

In the crucible of medical residency, where knowledge is tested, skills honed, and character forged, aspiring doctors embark on a transformative journey that will shape their professional lives forever.

From the halls of renowned hospitals to the bedside encounters with patients, the residency experience is a pivotal chapter in the saga of medical education.

It is a time of intense learning, profound growth, and relentless dedication as you navigate the intricate balance between clinical excellence, emotional resilience, and personal well-being.

In this book, you will delve into the intricate tapestry of the medical residency, exploring its challenges, triumphs, and the profound impact it has on those who dare to tread its path.

"The Journey through residency is tough, but the transformation it brings is priceless."

Chapter 1

HOW TO CHOOSE A SPECIALTY?

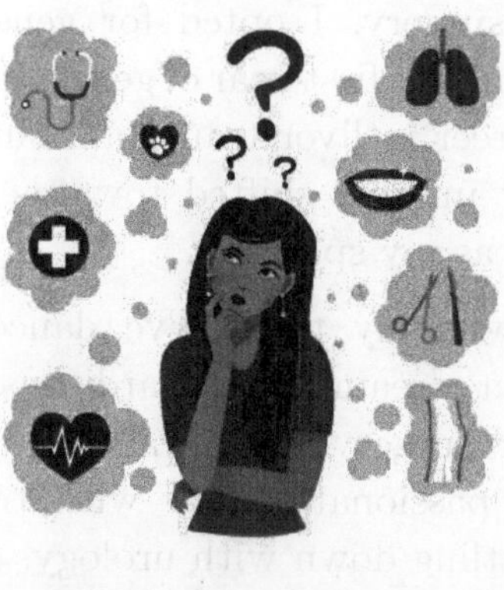

A question that troubles many once they secure a rank in NEET PG. You will see each week, your friends are switching their preferred branches for post-graduation studies. For example, someone who initially aimed for MS Orthopaedics is now considering MD Radiology, while another friend who planned on MD Medicine is now leaning towards MD Dermatology. After the merit list is released, there's typically about a month to finalize our post-graduate specialization choice. Much like seeking advice before exams, we turn to our seniors for invaluable insights into different branches. This pivotal decision often hinges on another person's experience and perspective of on a particular specialization. Coaching classes often organize counseling sessions where specialists from various branches discuss their field and the opportunities it offers. While many can outline the opportunities within their field, it's crucial to understand the underlying reasons behind choosing a specific branch.

Let me share how I've navigated my residency choices. Since middle school, I've aspired to become a surgeon, although initially, I wasn't sure which specialty or sub-specialty. Throughout medical school, my focus shifted from cardiovascular surgery to neurosurgery and then to gastrointestinal surgery. I opted for general surgery as a foundation. During my first year of general surgery residency, I aimed for a career in liver transplant surgery, but by the second year, my interest shifted towards urology, which I eventually chose as my specialty.

You see how many times I've danced with different specialties! From dreaming of cardiovascular surgery to flirting with neurosurgery, then swaying towards GI surgery, only to have a passionate affair with transplant surgery before finally settling down with urology.

Why?

As time progressed, I came to understand my genuine preferences and where my talents truly lie. Back then, the idea of becoming a CTVS or Heart Surgeon was merely a fantasy. Enthralled by the bravery and expertise portrayed in movies and books, I held heart surgeons in the highest regard. However, as I matured, I realized that my admiration for them was more about their courage and skill than a genuine desire to pursue that path.

Upon entering MBBS and completing my first year, the intricacies of neuroanatomy and its associated surgeries captivated my interest, igniting a fervent desire to pursue neurosurgery as my ultimate goal. This inclination was further fueled by the numerous residents at BJMC, Pune, who transitioned into neurosurgery following their MS in General Surgery. Their tales of excitement surrounding craniotomies resonated deeply with me.

As time went by and I wrapped up my final year of medical school, my interest veered towards GI surgery, armed with a solid theoretical foundation in general surgery. Joining my MS program at LTMMC, Sion, I found myself drawn to the world of liver transplantation. And what sparked this newfound fascination, you might ask? Well, I have Quora to thank for that. Dr. Vinay Kumaran, a Liver Transplant Surgeon, whose engaging presence and insightful contributions on Quora, as well as along with his career trajectory online, ignited a fresh ambition within me to pursue a career in liver transplantation. By my 2nd year of MS, I had gained a deeper comprehension of the field. Armed with knowledge about the various subspecialties, including the surgeries they perform, their lifestyle, job satisfaction, patient load, and working hours, I ultimately decided that urology was the perfect fit for me.

Were these decisions a walk in the park? Far from it. What made the journey smoother was the fire of my own knowledge and understanding. At first, my specialty picks were swayed by the perspectives of others. Yet, as I delved deeper, I unearthed a path that resonated with my own drive, hunger for growth, skill set, and heartfelt ambitions and aspirations in life.

"Choosing blindly based on limited understanding is akin to walking blindly into a minefield."

Now, let's delve into the process of acquiring the necessary knowledge to make this critical decision.

How do you determine which medical specialty suits you best? Do you select based on your interest in a specific organ or anatomical system? Or do you base your decision on whether you prefer to have extensive interaction with patients in primary care or minimal contact? Choosing a medical specialty is best done when you have a clear understanding of your own personality and temperament.

Deciding on a specialty is similar to the complex equations you've been working on throughout your adult life. It's a more intricate version of A + B = C. You can approach the decision-making process by breaking it down into logical steps to reach a well-informed conclusion.

A. What is Your Medical Practice Temperament?

You're more likely to be satisfied in your professional life if your career matches your interests, values, personality, and skills. To find your fit, first explore who you are and what you want for your life, then identify those career options that will support those goals.

B. Which Clinical Practice Scenarios Align With Your Traits?

Pace: Do you prefer handling emergency cases or a more predictable patient panel?

Severity: Do you enjoy managing critically ill patients regularly or would you rather deal with lower acuity cases?

Adrenaline: Do you thrive on the rush of trauma surgery and emergency patients, or do you prefer the more relaxed environment of primary care.

Lifestyle: Is maintaining your lifestyle more important to you than becoming the top physician in your field?

Patient interaction: Do you like interacting with patients like physicians/surgeons or you see yourself happy being in a paraclinical branch like Radiology/Pathology?

C. Walk a Mile in a Resident's Shoes?

Although many interns focus on studying and preparing for entrance exams, it's beneficial to spend time engaging with your residents during your internship. Develop relationships and inquire about their lifestyle, eating habits, emergency duties, and challenges they encounter in residency. Spend a full week working alongside them as the most junior resident to gain a clearer understanding of whether you'd enjoy the three years of residency if you had to join the department as a resident.

D. Prestige, Social Status & Social Expectations

The major dilemma in India revolves around choosing from medical specialties, which include prestige, status and financial rewards.

Example 1: Raj's father is a surgeon, but Raj prefers internal medicine. Although Raj has the opportunity to follow in his father's surgical footsteps, he opts for internal medicine, causing disappointment among his parents and extended family.

Example 2: Heta comes from a business-oriented family that wants her to specialize in MD Radiology so they can open a chain of diagnostic centers. However, Heta is more interested in pursuing Psychiatry as her specialty.

Example 3: Ram, who comes from a low-income family, has excelled in his medical education and wants to specialize in radiology. His family, who see surgeons and physicians as the most prestigious types of doctors, prefer he pursues MD Medicine.

You can envision countless scenarios, many of which you've likely experienced yourself. The question of whether a particular specialty offers more prestige or financial rewards than another will inevitably linger in your mind.

Choosing your specialty should be a personal decision. Focus on the areas of medicine where you feel the most fulfilled, and set aside how others—be it family, friends, or colleagues—who might judge your choice. Remember, every type of doctor plays a crucial role in the broader scope of medicine, and the notion that one specialty is more esteemed than another is subjective.

As medical students, who have excelled academically, it can be tough to shift away from always aiming to be the best. For some, fields like family practice or psychiatry may not seem as prestigious as being a world-renowned neurosurgeon or securing a spot in cardiology. However, as an emerging doctor, you no longer need to prove your worth to others.

By disregarding external pressures like social prestige and the expectations of others, you are more likely to select the specialty that's truly right for you, leading to a more satisfying and rewarding medical career.

E. Lifestyle Considerations

Medicine has consistently been a challenging profession. After putting in long hours at the hospital or clinic, physicians and surgeons often find themselves responding to calls in the middle of the night to deliver a baby, perform an emergency appendectomy, or admit a patient. Fed up with delayed gratification and unpredictable schedules, many doctors-in-training today seek careers that provide room for other interests or allow more time for their families. Modern medical students strive for a better work-life balance than past generations of physicians. They seek fewer night shifts, reduced hospital hours, and greater control over their work schedules.

What explains the increased focus on quality of life in medical careers? In the past, delayed gratification and nonstop hard work were the norms, shaping residency programs accordingly. However, the new generation of medical professionals wants to spend more time with their families and prioritizes a better quality of life.

For many current students, medicine, which was once viewed as a noble profession and a path to financial stability, now seems like a stressful and underpaid job. Instead of focusing solely on good patient care, today's resident has to cope with more paperwork, overnight phone calls from patients, loss of autonomy due to managed care, and the ever-growing threat of malpractice litigation and attacks by patients' relatives.

The so-called lifestyle specialties that the most academically successful students choose include Radiology & Dermatology, which allow you to control the number of hours you devote to your practice. You could potentially have a career with adequate family and leisure time, less stress, a more regular schedule, and an income commensurate with the workload; eventually it's a combination of what lifestyle you want. I wanted a busy lifestyle with adrenaline rush, patient interaction, use of new technology and minimal access surgeries; I chose Urology. Choose the lifestyle wisely!

F. Length of Training

Remember that different specialties require varying lengths of residency training. Generally, the shortest programs are at the end branches. MD Medicine and MS General Surgery offer super-specializations that add further training and an additional NEET SS entrance exam.

If you aim to subspecialize, expect to commit additional years to a fellowship. For example, cardiologists undergo a total of 6 years of training before starting their practice (3 years for an MD or DNB in Internal Medicine, followed by a 3-year DM or DrNB in Cardiology). Some doctors pursue even further specialization, like a cardiologist who completes an extra fellowship year to become proficient in electrophysiology; or a Urologist might want to have fellowships in Uro-Oncology.

G. Job Opportunities and Future

When you complete your residency, you'll face the decision of how to establish your practice. While there are some aspects you can anticipate now, many questions won't be resolved until you determine whether you will settle in a first, second, or third-tier city. How much of subspecialisation will be needed to establish your practice? Have a baseline idea of your future settlement (Might not always possible).

H. Special Considerations for Women

India, as a developing nation, has diverse social customs and norms. Many women prefer to consult female doctors for their health concerns, making careers in fields such as gynecology and breast surgery as great options for women. Women who want to prioritize family time may find paraclinical specialties to be a good choice.

Ask yourself if you would handle yourself working well in a predominantly male environment. Some specialties, especially technical ones, can be male-dominated. This is especially true for surgery and its subspecialties. It's important to be aware that high levels of testosterone in the workplace can lead to inappropriate comments, gender bias, and even sexual harassment. In environments like the operating room, a persistent locker room culture can pressure female surgeons to conform to male behavior to fit in with their colleagues. Regardless of your specialty, it's crucial to feel comfortable with the physicians you work alongside. A supportive work environment is essential for both your well-being and the quality of patient care. Are you ready for this kind of work setting? Have an answer to these questions!

I. Passion

When it comes to choosing a medical specialty, the advice to "follow your passion" gets thrown around more than confetti at a parade. But let's be real: passion is one of the most overused and misused words out there. It's defined as a very strong feeling, especially of love, hate, or anger. I like urology and enjoy working in the field, but would I say I'm passionate about it? Probably not – that sounds like an exaggeration.

Nowadays, with hundreds of books and articles on career choices, it's easy to feel like you're missing out (FOMO) if you're not following some burning passion. When I watched "3 Idiots" as a kid, I believed everyone had a passion they should pursue, and that those who didn't were just slogging through life, miserably.

At 25, did I know my passion? Nope.

Do I know it now? Still no.

Will I find out what it is in the future? Beats me.

I might never find it, and that's okay.

So, don't beat yourself up just because someone else claims they've found their passion. It's perfectly fine if your job isn't your life's passion. Ask your parents if they've always been passionate about their professions. Odds are, they'll say no. At 25, I hadn't even performed a single surgery – how could I be passionate about something I'd never done? How can anyone know what they're passionate about without trying out different specialties?

Instead of chasing after the latest buzzword, focus on gaining insight into various specialties. Make your decision based on experience, not hype. Who knows, you might just find that you enjoy urology – or something else entirely – without the need for fireworks and confetti.

Making the Decision

How important is each factor? You should answer for yourself. What is important for you may not be as important for your friends and family helping you make a decision. Try to give it a score based on your own preferences. If lifestyle is more important to you than the length of training then give lifestyle more points. Add your points and then choose from the top 3.

As you dive into the decision-making abyss of your medical journey, remember this; whether you're choosing cardiology or neurology, you're basically adding one more doctor to the mix who just wants to make the world a tad healthier.

> ***"Choosing a medical specialty is like trying to pick your favorite symptom—impossible and slightly absurd, but hey, at least you'll always have a story for cocktail parties!"***

Chapter 2

HOW TO CHOOSE A RESIDENCY PROGRAM?

So you've chosen a specialty, or atleast narrowed down to a few. Now selecting a residency program is an exhilarating journey akin to choosing your specialty! It's a pivotal moment that sets the stage for your medical career. Dive in early, explore your options, and gather insights from diverse sources to find the perfect match. Get ready to embark on an adventure where your educational goals meet endless opportunities for growth and fulfillment!

Gathering Information:

1. Seats available in your specialty
2. Location: Cities and states
3. Rank cut-off for that particular residency program
4. Facilities available; Hostels, Labs
5. Faculty and workload
6. Colleagues
7. Academics
8. MD Vs DNB (DM/Mch Vs DrNB)
9. Government Vs Private
10. Stipend and Government bonds

1. Seats available in your specialty

This should be straightforward. You should be able to get this on NBE's official website. Each year, they add new residency programs at various institutions. Each year they update the matrix before counselling starts. Prior to the release just make a list as per previous years matrix and then readjust accordingly if new seats are added.

2. Location: Cities and States

Choose the locations you would like to go. There will be 50% seat filling via state counselling and 50% via national counselling. Have a general idea on where you want to go. Specific issues faced in India like language, stipend, state bond, travel time to hometown, relatives, familiarity to weather, etc. will matter.

3. Rank cut-off for that particular residency program

In selecting my residency program, I compiled a spreadsheet that details the past three years of counseling sessions (typically 2-3 rounds) for both state and national programs. This provided a rapid assessment of the average rank required for specific institutions. State lists often favor residents from the respective state.

4. Facilities available: Hostels, Labs

Once you've identified potential institutions, initiate inquiries with current residents regarding accommodations (Hostel vs. Wards), laboratory amenities, Modular Operating Rooms, Surgical Intensive Care Units (SICUs), state-of-the-art surgical equipment (such as laparoscopic instruments, lasers, endoscopes), Trauma wards and medical facilities like ICU beds, Neonatal ICUs (NICUs), Pediatric ICUs (PICUs), etc.

5. Faculty and workload

One of the crucial inquiries revolves around identifying the mentors who will guide you throughout your residency. Engage with multiple current residents to gain a comprehensive understanding of the department's faculty members. Explore the department's culture and norms. Inquire about the routine responsibilities assigned to residents, any additional duties expected, and the workload dynamics such as patient volume in wards, Outpatient Departments (OPD), Inpatient Department (IPD) admissions, patient turnover rates, number of emergency duties, ICU postings, trauma duties, health camps, superspeciality exposure and the extent of hands-on surgical experience for surgical residents. Delve into their typical week's schedule to gain deeper insights into the residency experience.

Understanding the resident-to-unit ratio and whether there is unit rotation throughout the academic year is crucial information. Inquire about the number of residents in the institution and how they are distributed among units. Assess if unit rotation is implemented and how units are allocated, particularly in terms of ranking or other criteria. This ensures a balanced consideration between being in the optimal unit within a second-choice institution versus being in a less favorable unit within a first-choice institution.

It's essential to sniff out any departmental or institutional "toxicity" before diving in headfirst. After all, you want to know who you'll be rubbing elbows with every day. I cannot emphasis enough on this aspect. This would probably be more important than you think.

You should be interested in asking about interns! Are interns at that institution completing their internship rotations throughout the year, or they are like a rare sighting in the wild and all appear in a grand flock after entrance exams, completing their internships on paper en masse? And the legendary resident-intern couples, the real-life medical drama that puts Grey's Anatomy to shame! We all know someone! Apart from all the serious stuff (work), make sure to sneak in some gossip from interns, the juicy details that keep the hospital corridors buzzing!

6. Colleagues

Identify individuals with similar residency preferences and comparable ranks, then engage in thorough discussions to dissect potential scenarios and share insightful analyses. Through this collaborative process, you may uncover prospective residency colleagues who align with your professional trajectory.

7. Academics

Examine the academic caliber within the department, scrutinizing aspects such as case discussions, grand rounds, presentations, journal clubs, paper presentations, publications, and participation in conferences. Academic prowess can delineate the distinction between an average and an exemplary physician.

8. MD/MS Vs DNB (DM/MCh Vs DrNB)

The enduring debate over the equivalence of DNB and MD is a testament to the multifaceted nature of medical education. Having pursued MS General Surgery followed by DrNB Urology, I deliberated over opting for MCh and ultimately chose a different path as my priorities evolved. My MS training, entrenched within one of India's most bustling General Surgery residency programs, provided invaluable lessons. However, for my superspeciality journey, I yearned for greater exposure to private healthcare settings with state-of-the-art facilities and patients from higher socioeconomic backgrounds and similar workload to government institutions. I was disinclined towards the additional governmental bond commitments (2-3 years) that MCh entailed.

While MD/MS from government setups offers an unparalleled experience; sleeping in ward side rooms, grappling with equipment shortages, racing through wards for blood collections, and navigating bureaucratic hurdles; it fosters a profound sense of humility and gratitude, enriching one's perspective on life immeasurably.

I'm biased towards advocating for experiencing both worlds, but hey, it's all about personal preference! The key is to make an informed decision. Perceived prestige may vary, some individuals may consider DNB degrees to have less acclaim compared to MD degrees earned from esteemed institutions. I could sit and discuss about all the pros and cons but I would refrain as its a personal choice. I preferred MS followed by DrNB. I thank myself enough for making these decisions. I sloughed through my MS and developed raw surgical and communication skills & now I have a more balanced work with supervised hands on where my surgical skills are honed by the best in the field. My communication has improved with more educated class of patients, who need detailed explanation of the disease and expected course of disease.

9. Government Vs Private

Private residency programs in medical institutions often provide access to modern facilities, exposure to patients from higher socioeconomic backgrounds, and lower salaries for residents. However, they may lack the diverse patient population and extensive hands-on experience seen in government institutions. On the other hand, government residency programs offer valuable exposure to a wide range of cases, opportunities to serve diverse communities, and typically come with fewer financial burdens for residents. However, they may face resource constraints and bureaucratic challenges. The choice between private and government residency programs ultimately depends on individual preferences, career goals, and financial considerations.

10. Stipend and Government bonds

In the realm of medical residency, the initial stipend often serves as the primary source of income for individuals, many of whom are between the ages of 24 and 30. Despite being in the midst of educational pursuits and degree acquisition, the financial aspect remains crucial, particularly for those seeking autonomy from parental support or considering marriage. In India, remuneration varies across states, ranging from Rs. 40,000 to Rs. 1,10,000 accentuating the significance of financial considerations during this pivotal phase of professional development.

Another significant concern is the government bond requirement imposed by each state, which typically ranges from 1 to 5 years. It's crucial to recognize that these bonds can either impede professional advancement or, conversely, provide opportunities for growth, depending on individual circumstances.

Example 1: Consider the case of Dr. Sameer, aged 31, hailing from Madhya Pradesh. Having completed his MBBS, MS in General Surgery, and MCh in Neurosurgery in Maharashtra, he finds himself with a substantial bond obligation of 4 years. This duration comprises 1 year for MBBS, 1 year for MS, and 2 years for MCh. Should he opt to practice in Madhya Pradesh, he faces the dilemma of either fulfilling the remaining 4 years in Maharashtra or paying a hefty sum of almost Rs. 1.6 crores (10 lakhs + 50 lakhs + 1 crore) to terminate his bonds prematurely. In hindsight, he might have made a more advantageous decision by pursuing his SS in DrNB (Instead of Mch) and MS in Madhya Pradesh, thereby saving 3 years of bond commitment in Maharashtra, equivalent to 1.5 crores. The complexities of bond agreements, often overlooked in one's early twenties, can yield frustration and distress for young professionals. It underscores the importance of gaining a preliminary understanding of such contractual obligations before embarking on a career path, given the significant impact that a 4-year commitment can have on one's trajectory.

Example 2: Dr. Neha, a 28-year-old doctor, who recently completed her MD in Anaesthesia, faces a unique situation. Having obtained both her MBBS and MD Anaesthesia degrees in Maharashtra, she is now married and thinking of her professional trajectory. With a bond commitment of 2 years, she seeks to accrue valuable experience in a bustling government healthcare environment, initially as a Senior Resident, with aspirations of eventually transitioning to an Assistant Professor role. The government bond offers her the opportunity to engage in this career progression, ensuring a consistent monthly income while honing her skills and expertise within the public healthcare system.

In the intricate maze of the Indian healthcare system, I've witnessed colleagues resort to some creative maneuvering just to dodge those pesky bonds. It's like watching a scene from a medical themed sitcom; doctors juggling between private colleges, DNB/DrNB programs, and a side dish of existential crisis, all to avoid being shackled to a government bond.

Mastering the intricacies of healthcare education in India is crucial; some excel at navigating its complexities, while others find themselves overwhelmed by the system's demands.

Chapter 3

PREPARING FOR RESIDENCY

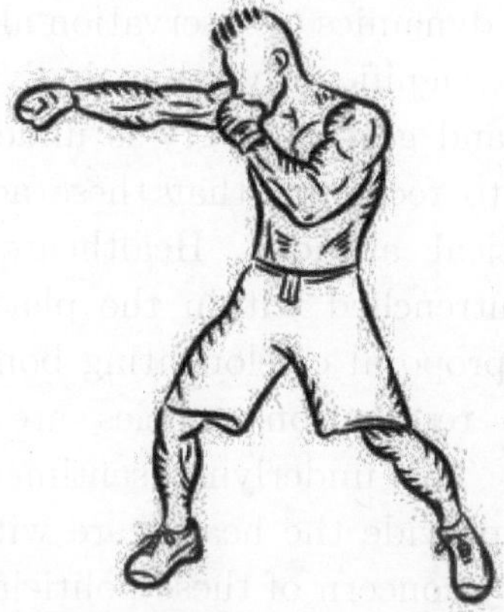

Alright, buckle up for the rollercoaster ride of the next few years after locking in your branch and institution preferences. Get ready to play the waiting game because every year, like clockwork, some state government decides to throw a wrench in the works by filing a case, delaying counseling sessions by a good 1-2 months. And oh, let's not forget the thrilling plot twists of reservation changes driven by political dramas! It's enough to make even the calmest person want to pull their hair out, or maybe even join the circus instead of dealing with this counseling circus!

Ah, the sage advice in the midst of chaos: Keep Calm and Carry On, even when the rumor mill is working overtime, churning out misinformation faster than a street food vendor on a busy day. Get ready to dive headfirst into those random Telegram and WhatsApp groups, where paying to fight a case becomes the latest trend, because why not? And who can resist the temptation to flood NBE with calls? We are a mere pawn in the political game of healthcare hot potato. The judiciary will observe with vacation during the summer and Diwali periods, keeping the cases pending in the courts.

The intricate dynamics of reservation alterations possess the potential to significantly alter individuals' rankings and preferences and getting angry is understandable. Yet, it is imperative to recognize that these adjustments often align with political agendas. Healthcare, a cornerstone issue, remains entrenched within the platforms of myriad politicians. The proposal of elongating bond durations and modifications to reservation policies are promises made during elections. The underlying sentiment of welfare of individuals who provide the healthcare within this context is not the primary concern of these politicians.

To some extent we live in a bubble where its easy to be swept away by believing that everything has stopped because 100,000 MBBS graduates are awaiting counselling! People don't care. Apart from a few of your closest family members and friends, no one cares! Society sees doctors as privileged! It may be tempting to perceive ourselves as significant, particularly when bombarded with impassioned blogs and lengthy online posts detailing the plight of over 100,000 MBBS graduates awaiting court rulings, confined to their homes. However, it is crucial to maintain perspective within the broader context of India's staggering population exceeding 140 crores. In the eyes of these politicians, individuals embroiled in such circumstances are likely viewed as privileged exceptions rather than focal points of concern.

So it right on the government's part to delay counselling each year? NO, absolutely not. But it will likely happen. Here are some things you'd rather focus on during this drama.

1. Improve your health: Embarking on residency is an exhilarating journey for both body and mind. Embrace the pre-residency time as an opportunity to incorporate exercise into your routine, whether it's hitting the gym, engaging in outdoor workouts, or indulging in your favorite sports. It's natural to experience weight fluctuations during preparations, but don't be fooled into thinking that residency will automatically shed those extra pounds. Remember, sustainable weight loss is the key to a healthy lifestyle. Prioritize regular exercise before residency kicks off to boost your overall well-being and keep your mind blissfully occupied, steering clear of the counseling drama. Plus, who can resist the daily dose of endorphins that come with staying active?

2. Spend time with your loved ones: Treasure these precious 1-2 months as a gift of time bestowed upon you to cherish moments with your dear MBBS friends and beloved family members. As you prepare to embark on the intense journey of residency, embrace the opportunity to immerse yourself in the warmth of companionship and familial bonds. In the whirlwind of the upcoming 3 years, you'll inevitably drift apart from many of your undergraduate friends, and visits home will become rare occurrences, spaced out over months. So, let the embrace of friendship and love envelop you now, filling your heart with memories to carry you through the challenges ahead. Retrospectively I can see I have missed so many weddings; many of them were my best friends.

3. Hobbies: Nurture your hobbies to manage stress during residency. Whether it's painting, dancing, singing, or anything else you enjoy.

4. Travel: Extended leaves can be challenging during residency. If you enjoy traveling, take the opportunity to go on treks or road trips. However, ensure you stay within network. Counseling details might be released unexpectedly.

5. Family: Some of you come from families with dozens of doctors & some of you will be the 1st doctor in the family. A key difference here will be preparing your family for your residency. Not picking up phones, seeing parents once in 6 months, sudden weight loss, unable to attend every family function or a cousin's wedding, etc.

For students originating from medical lineages, these situations are all too familiar to their parents and relatives. They find solace in simply being in your presence, gladly accommodating your need for rest during gatherings, and offering unwavering support during challenging phases of your residency journey. I still remember how comforting my family members were during my MS, whenever I would meet or talk with them.

For those destined to be the inaugural doctors in their families, conveying the realities of their lives can be an arduous task. Parents and relatives might express disappointment over missed calls or absenteeism from significant events like weddings. Questions about sudden weight loss or perpetual fatigue can further strain these interactions. Conversations with family members unacquainted with the rigors of residency can prove challenging, with the desire for familial support sometimes met with accusations of arrogance or self-absorption. The journey of pioneering into medicine can evoke a sense of profound isolation and sadness as the demands of residency erode the foundation of family connections. The toll is heavy: missed calls from worried loved ones, rare visits home, a fading presence at family gatherings, and the heartache of absenting oneself from cherished celebrations like weddings.

Initiating a heartfelt dialogue with your parents and close relatives is crucial to prepare them for the journey ahead. By explaining that your residency demands will require periods of absence and sacrifice, you're laying the groundwork for their understanding and support. Emphasize that while you may not always be physically present, their unwavering encouragement and understanding are invaluable as you navigate the challenges of residency. These conversations serve as anchors, ensuring that despite the physical distance, your familial bonds remain steadfast and resilient as you dedicate yourself to your medical career.

I can't stress this enough. Many of my friends from non-medical backgrounds struggled to explain why they hadn't spoken in 3-4 days or why they seemed in such a hurry to end phone calls. Their families might even joke that they had joined a war, given how busy they always were! I recall a friend feeling disheartened when he saw me having a brief, two-minute conversation with my parents, untroubled by emotional appeals about my absence. In contrast, every one of his calls would be met with a barrage of emotional pleas.

To Mom & Dad

In heartfelt talks, with coffee in hand,
Explain the plan, help them understand.
Residency's wild, you'll be MIA,
Not just lazy, or on holiday.

"Mom, Dad, I'll miss many dinners," you say,
"No, I'm not avoiding you this way."
My absence is tough, not just a quirk,
Though I might text from the depths of my
hospital work.

Their support's gold, a priceless treasure,
Even when they guilt-trip for good measure.
"We'll miss you, but we get it, dear,"
"Just send a photo from the hospital, we'll
cheer!"

Conversations keep bonds tight and true,
Despite your vanishing act, they'll see you
through.
So laugh it off, and keep them near,
In residency's madness, their love will cheer.

Dr. Alhad Naragude

Section – B

What To Expect during Residency?

Chapter 4

THE RESIDENCY

Who is a Resident Doctor?

The term "resident doctor" has historical roots in the development of modern medical education. In the early 20th century, medical education underwent significant reforms in the United States, moving away from apprenticeship-based training to structured programs with defined curriculum and supervised clinical experience. As part of these reforms, newly graduated physicians would live and work in hospitals under the guidance of experienced faculty members, hence the term "resident" to signify their presence within the hospital. Over time, residency training became a crucial phase of medical education, providing doctors with hands-on experience and specialized training in their chosen field. Today, residency programs are an integral part of medical training globally, and the term "resident doctor" is widely recognized to refer to physicians undergoing postgraduate training.

Upon embarking on your residency program, it's likely you'll be granted a few weeks to acclimate to both the new city surroundings and the hospital environment.

For many clinical specialties, the ward sideroom becomes your primary residence. As the go-to resident for ward matters, allow yourself time to adjust; it's a challenging transition. Embrace this fresh start as you familiarize yourself with the hospital's infrastructure, from labs to operating rooms, blood banks to radiology facilities. Forge connections with fellow residents across departments; these new friendships not only ease the adjustment but also streamline your reference processes. Radiology, Microbiology, and Pathology friends become invaluable allies for residents in clinical branches.

Basic duties that you'll start doing will include:

1. Conducting ongoing evaluations of patients' states.

2. Reviewing patient backgrounds and conducting physical assessments.

3. Supporting physicians during their regular rounds.

4. Documenting observations, generating reports, and composing discharge summaries.

5. Initiating test and medication requests.

6. Interacting with patients and their families, articulating diagnoses clearly, and outlining treatment strategies.

7. Handling critical situations and emergencies.

8. Radiology residents will start observing ultrasounds, CT Scans, writing reports, giving emergency appointments.

9. Pathology and microbiology residents start basics as per their postings in various subdivisions.

Additionally, residents often participate in teaching medical students and other healthcare professionals. Their responsibilities vary depending on their level of training and the specific requirements of their residency program and specialty. While these might be the basic expectations from you, most of us find ourselves doing a lot more than these. Here are some things you'll do irrespective of whether its a part of your duty or not.

1. Investigations: Ask any resident in a clinical branch, and they'll tell you that arranging investigations for patients often falls on the shoulders of the most junior resident in the department. You'll often find yourself pleading for CT or ultrasound appointments or rushing to the laboratory with your patient's blood sample to get a CBC done. If you're in Radiology or Pathology, accepting requests from colleagues for lab tests or emergency CT scan appointments at late hours might earn you bashing from seniors.

Labs and radiology departments may argue that investigations are being overused, while clinicians stress the importance of thoroughness to avoid overlooking any potential issues. As a new resident, it's important not to take everything said by your seniors to heart, as you may find yourself aligned with either side in the above debate!

2. Finances: In many institutions, there are social workers available to assist patients with financial concerns, providing support for accessing expensive medications or investigations not provided by the institution free of charge. As a resident, you'll often collaborate with these social workers to ensure your patients receive the necessary treatment. I still remember the innumerable visits to Sunday friends (Charity Organisation) at LTMMC, Sion.

3. MPW (Multipurpose Workers): In many government hospitals, residents often find themselves multitasking, from pushing trolleys to running blood investigations due to a shortage of technicians, shifting patients, handling crowds, and even cleaning OT tables. This additional workload can be incredibly frustrating, with little action taken despite complaints to higher-ups or departments. Eventually, residents often resign themselves to accepting it, as battling bureaucracy can feel like a futile endeavor. Your grievances often encounter responses along the lines of, "Back in our day as residents, things were far more challenging."

Such challenges are less common in private hospitals or privately funded institutions (DNB/DrNB) & lately has been a key factor in residents opting these institutions over government institutions. (It scores more points while they analyse what residency to choose). If it is an important criterion for you, you should also weigh the pros and cons accordingly.

As you reflect on this, let it inspire rather than discourage you. When I began my residency, I embraced the workload with readiness and enthusiasm. Through the additional responsibilities, such as managing with limited resources and advocating for financial assistance for patients, I gained invaluable lessons. I discovered the importance of financial management firsthand and developed a knack for multitasking, from running labs to maneuvering equipment in the OT without technicians. Even tasks like cleaning the OT became opportunities for learning and growth. This optimistic outlook allowed me to understand the system better and focus my energy on personal growth and learning rather than dwelling on its flaws. Embrace each challenge as a chance to learn and improve; it's a mindset that fosters resilience and fuels progress.

4. Communication: Throughout your residency, the aspect poised for the most significant growth is undoubtedly communication skills! Residency marks your inaugural foray into a professional setting, where you're not just a student anymore; you're an employee with a stipend and assigned basic responsibilities. It's a dynamic environment where your ability to communicate effectively with colleagues at all levels of the hierarchy is thoroughly put to the test.

In residency, the days of dodging crucial communication are behind you! Now, you're thrust into situations where effective interaction is non-negotiable. Whether you're a fan of everyone around you or not, you'll find yourself needing to communicate with them. Embrace it! As you climb the residency ladder, you'll discover the art of not just getting work done but also adeptly managing the workplace and its people.

Reminiscing about what my unit head once quoted during my final year of residency: **"The third year of your residency is akin to earning an MBA—you'll master the art of managing everything around you. From the OT list to patient discharges, from overseeing juniors and their duties to being the scapegoat for any management mishaps!** It's like being in a crash course of business management, only with more adrenaline and fewer law suits!"

Discovering the importance of patience in communication was truly eye-opening! During my first residency, amidst the chaos of overwhelming patient volumes and bureaucratic hurdles, patience was a rare commodity. 200 patients in OPD seen by 6-7 doctors in 3-4 hours! Most of the patients received limited explainations. Now in my 2nd residency where patient management is smoother and resources abound, I learned that I lacked patience. Over the first few months engaging in conversations with patients and their families for up to 15 minutes, addressing their concerns and clearing doubts, became a rewarding journey of empathy and understanding and improved my patience! Each of you will enter residency with different level of ability to communicate, but most of you will upgrade your communication skills.

5. Stock bag: In a government hospital setting, a significant responsibility entails maintaining an inventory of essential instruments, central lines, dressing materials, bandages, sutures, discharge summary templates, requisition letters, SpO_2 probes, stethoscopes, and more. This unique aspect of the Government Residency Program may not always be met with enthusiasm; frustrations with government bureaucracy or resource availability may arise. Nevertheless, residents are entrusted with the task of managing the stock bag, ensuring that necessary supplies are readily accessible. In times of need, any item unavailable in the wards is expected to be replenished from this stock. Even your unit heads are aware of stock bags! So keeping it refilled is a duty handed over to the 1st year & overseen by 2nd year resident.

6. Workload: The workload in medical residency can vary greatly depending on your specialty and the institution you are affiliated with. It's a well-known phenomenon that senior residents often boast about the extensive hours they've worked, and they might even claim that the current juniors are not as hard-working as they were. This sentiment is quite universal—every generation seems to feel that the following one has it easier. It's all a matter of perspective.

For instance, I knew that I could handle working 18-20 hours a day. Some of my colleagues managed very well for 15-18 hours but found it challenging beyond 18 hours. The question arises: did the ability to work for longer made me a better resident? If your instinctive answer is yes, you might want to reconsider. Every individual has their own capacity and endurance. Working 18 hours a day equates to 126 hours over the course of a week. How could someone working these many hours possibly be considered a poor resident? Even those who work 15 hours a day are putting in 105 hours a week. This is more than double the recommended 48-hour work week. Everyone has their capacity; remember that doesn't make you a bad resident.

The notion of working long hours as a badge of honor is deeply ingrained in the medical profession. It's a game of endurance and resilience, but it also raises important questions about the quality of patient care, the well-being of the residents, and the overall efficiency of the healthcare system.

From my experience, being able to work extensive hours doesn't necessarily correlate with being a better resident. The quality of the work performed, the ability to make sound decisions under pressure, and maintain a compassionate attitude towards patients are equally, if not more important. Working beyond one's capacity can lead to burnout, reduced cognitive function, and ultimately, compromises in patient care.

Historically, medical training has included rigorous hours, and this culture of medicine has often celebrated this as a rite of passage. However, this tradition is increasingly being questioned and will probably have better outcomes in the future. Critics of duty hour restrictions argue that the limitations hinder the training process and do not allow residents to see through complex cases from start to finish. They believe that the experience gained during these long hours is invaluable and irreplaceable. The debate over the appropriate number of working hours for residents is not just a matter of personal endurance but also touches upon the broader issues of healthcare delivery and medical education. The issue of resident workload is also tied to the overall structure and efficiency of the healthcare system. Hospitals that rely heavily on residents working long hours may be masking deeper systemic issues, such as understaffing or inefficient processes. Addressing these root causes could lead to more sustainable solutions that do not rely on exhausting residents.

Before committing to any specialty and institution, it's crucial to do thorough research. Ultimately, the key is to learn and adapt to the system around you to become more efficient. This debate about working hours will persist. Keep in mind that struggling to work 18-20 hours a day does not mean you will become a bad doctor.

7. Interpersonal relations: Interpersonal relations in a medical residency are critical to both personal well-being and professional development.

Team Dynamics: Residents often work in teams/units, including attending physicians, fellow residents, nurses, and other healthcare professionals. Residents rely heavily on mentorship from attending physicians and senior residents. Establishing a respectful and open relationship with mentors can enhance learning experiences.

Peer Relationships: Interactions with fellow residents can provide emotional support and camaraderie, which are vital given the demanding nature of residency. Building a supportive network can help manage stress and prevent burnout. However, competition and comparison can sometimes strain these relationships, so fostering a cooperative rather than competitive environment is beneficial. In an environment where everyone is overworked; showing empathy could help you understand the challenges.

Imagine needing an urgent CT scan, only to have your request denied by the Radiology resident, who is not only your friend but also your batchmate. Their refusal isn't personal; it's because their senior has given strict instructions. As a first-year resident, you're bound by a hierarchy, too. Instead of escalating into a fight over the CT scan, try to understand their position and communicate your reasons clearly. Expressing the urgency and importance of the scan, and conveying this effectively, can help both parties reach a resolution without conflict. This approach fosters empathy and collaboration, essential for navigating the complexities of medical residency. This also holds true for 2D echo, blood banks, ANC scans, etc.

8. Conflicts: Conflicts are inevitable in the high-stress environment of medical residencies, especially when exhaustion and heavy workloads are part of daily life. Imagine 2 sleep deprived residents clashing in the ER over who should manage a patient with a diabetic foot. Surgery plans to amputate the toe and expects Medicine to handle the Diabetic Ketoacidosis (DKA), while Medicine insists the patient should be admitted under Surgery, as the DKA is infection-related. This sparks a heated argument.

Such fights over patient admissions between Surgery and Medicine are legendary, with both sides often at fault. Knowing these weekly ER confrontations were inevitable, my co-junior residents from Medicine and I decided to forge a pact. We agreed that if a case ultimately needed surgery, we would take the patient, and if it was a medical issue, they would handle it. We synchronized our emergency days and corresponding medical units for an entire year. This arrangement worked wonders, quelling the long-standing rivalry that plagued our senior batches. Our solution highlighted the critical role of communication and cooperation.

In high-pressure settings like this, mastering conflict resolution is essential. Recognizing issues early, appreciating different perspectives, and finding mutually acceptable solutions can transform a combative atmosphere into one of collaboration. Eventually both sides are overworked; atleast this way you're not bothered by managing patient where your experience and expertise is lacking.

The Alliance

In the ER's turmoil, two tired souls clash,
Over a diabetic foot, tensions dash.
Surgery eyes the toe, ready to amend,
While Medicine insists, DKA to tend.

Patient's fate hangs in the heated air,
Admissions debated, with flair.
Legends of clashes, each side keen,
Weekly confrontations, stormy scene.

Co-juniors from Medicine, a pact we made,
To ease the chaos that ERs parade.
Synchronized days and units aligned,
For a year, peace in our minds entwined.

For when surgery calls, Medicine yields,
And when medical woes, Surgery shields.
A pact forged in ER's nightly throng,
Where teamwork triumphs, hearts stay
strong.

Dr. Alhad Naragude

9. Relatives & Violence: We all have heard and seen news articles about relatives going crazy bashing doctors after demise of their patients.

I'll recount a harrowing incident from my second year of residency. An elderly man with esophageal cancer, whose family had already been informed about his poor prognosis and the need for palliative care at home, was brought to the ER in a gasping state. My junior attended to him first, and upon being informed, I proceeded to intubate the patient. However, the situation quickly escalated. The patient's two sons, both visibly drunk, began causing a ruckus in the ER, despite the presence of security guards who merely watched from a distance. The elder son, fuming with rage, stood 2 feet away from me, shouting accusations as if I had caused his father's condition, while my junior ventilated the patient with an ambu bag.

The ER, already crowded with around 100 people attending to their own patients, became a hotspot. A murmur spread, and it seemed the crowd was ready to erupt into violence. Just then, my lecturer, familiar with the patient and his family from the OPD, arrived and explained the situation. The elder son grabbed my lecture's collar, demanding to know if his father would die. I stood barely a foot away from what felt like an inevitable assault. Within seconds, about 25-30 residents from all departments rushed in, and the police arrived to disperse the growing mob while security still stayed back, watching. What defused the immediate threat was my calm, polite response about the patient's status, despite the chaos. Was it the perfect solution? I don't know. Handling an emotionally charged mob, especially one from Dharavi, Mumbai, is unpredictable. I consider myself fortunate; had I shown any panic or pushed the aggressive relative, I might have ended up as another

Handling the Heat

In the unpredictable storm of a mob,
Even calm words may not do the job.
For residents, the wisest course,
Is to communicate the worst, at times with force.

Always prepare the kin for the worst,
Repeatedly, so their bubble bursts.
Will it guarantee your safety? Who can tell?
But it's a strategy that could serve you well.

Identify those who might react with rage,
Prepare them gently, at every stage.
In moments of heat, emotion reigns,
Their status won't matter, only their pains.

Involve your seniors, call for aid,
Hospital management, make sure they're played.
Proactive talk, strategic might,
Could prevent chaos from taking flight.

In this field where tensions run high,
This approach could be your ally.
For in the world of care and strife,
These steps might just protect your life.

Dr. Alhad Naragude

assaulted medical resident in the news. It's impossible to always remain calm during such incidents when you're overworked and sleep-deprived.

It's impossible to predict what a mob will do. Even if you stay calm, you might get hit just because the relatives are crazy! For residents, the best strategy is to always communicate the worst-case scenarios to the patient's relatives, emphasizing it every time you update them on the patient's condition. Will this guarantee your safety? You'll never know. But learning to identify troublesome relatives and preparing them for the worst is a wiser approach. In the heat of the moment, the relatives' educational status won't matter; they're driven by emotion. Always involve your seniors and hospital management when necessary. This proactive communication and strategic involvement might just be the key to preventing a volatile situation from spiraling out of control.

Academics

During residency, balancing academics, research, and thesis work is a daunting yet essential task for medical professionals. This period marks a crucial phase where you not only gain clinical expertise but also contribute to medical knowledge through research and academic pursuits. Amidst the demanding schedule of patient care and hospital rotations, you are also expected to engage in academic activities that foster your growth as a future physician and contribute to the advancement of medical science.

The role of research is a cornerstone of medical progress, fostering innovation and evidence-based practice.

Thesis or dissertation work: Most residency programs in India require a thesis or dissertation as a compulsory part of the training, mandatory before exams. However, how many of us genuinely engage with it, or even have an interest in it, has been a topic of debate for ages. During my final year, working on my thesis taught me how literature reviews and statistics are crucial in medical research. It provided me with a basic understanding of how to read scientific papers and helped me comprehend a particular disease more thoroughly. How thesis research is done in most places is well known to all residents and faculties.

We all face challenges during academic pursuits, and in Indian residencies, these challenges are the biggest deterrents to academic progress.

Time management: *Sonay ka time nahi hai, paper kab likhu?*

Work-life balance: If I find any free time, I'd rather sleep and eat well. Priorities!

Research funding: Almost nil. It's you, wandering around with no financial support, spending your own money on a statistician, and no one to help collect data.

Publication and presentation: Minimal understanding of how it's done. (Presenting your first paper is like climbing Everest, but it does get easier from there)

How many papers did I publish during my first residency? None. Was I interested? I wasn't sure. I picked a residency program famous for its hands-on learning, not its academic reputation. The focus was on operating and learning by doing, with minimal academic activities over three years. No one was keen on teaching academics, and residents were too swamped to care. I chose this residency to gain practical experience, and lack of academics didn't bother me. All of us passed MS with flying colors despite the minimal academic involvement. We attended zero CMEs or conferences.

Presenting the Findings

In residency's rush, amidst the grind,
A paper to present, with knowledge to find.
Late nights with charts, data to glean,
Hoping our findings will make a good scene.

Slides perfected, nerves held tight,
Presenting our research in academic light.
Questions arise, we stand our ground,
Sharing our work, where new insights are found.

With a sigh of relief, the task complete,
In the realm of research, we've claimed our seat.
A short victory in residency's fight,
Blending practice and research makes one shine bright.

Dr. Alhad Naragude

My first realization of the importance of academics came during my INI-SS interview for Urology. The first five minutes were all about academics—conferences, paper presentations, awards, etc. I aced the extracurricular section, chatting about football, badminton, and chess. After four spotter questions, my interview ended. I knew I had nailed three out of four.

Then, the crisis hit. Three years with no academic achievements to show! In a WhatsApp group of 30 surgeons prepping for the Urology interview, everyone had papers, urology experience, and SRships. I was just an MS passout with no academic credentials. Answering the urology questions well didn't matter—many others did too. I failed to get a good rank because of my lack of academic experience.

This was my first "aha" moment about the importance of academics. They make a big difference in interviews, fellowships, and future job opportunities. Now, understanding their significance in my career trajectory, I'm now making efforts to boost my academic accomplishments.

Exams: I remember when I started my residency, my brother advised me to read something every day. Did I follow his advice? No. Did he follow it in his residency? No. But hey, we all recommend it! It's probably easier said than done, especially in surgical branches where skill acquisition is emphasized more than book smarts.

You'll have exams, and trust me, you don't want to be overwhelmed by the mountain of books waiting for you. A small handbook of standard textbooks can make a huge difference in your theoretical understanding. Many guidelines and lectures are now available for free on the internet. A 10-minute lecture video on the go or watching a procedure on YouTube just to brush up can really boost your comfort and confidence levels. Everyone has their own learning style. Stick to yours and soak up as much knowledge as you can.

Chapter 5

MENTAL HEALTH

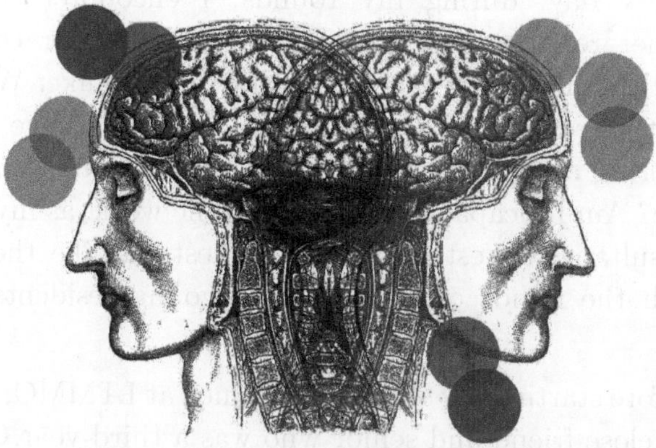

"You have been formed of 3 parts—body, breath, and mind. Of these, the first 2 are yours insofar as they are only in your care. The third alone is truly yours."

–Marcus Aurelius, Meditations

The body can suffer from disease, injury, or sudden disability. It can endure imprisonment or torture, and the breath can cease naturally or be taken forcefully. Breathing may become difficult due to exertion or illness. However, throughout it all, our mind remains our own. It's not that our body and breath, as Marcus Aurelius mentions, are insignificant. They are simply less under our complete control compared to our mind. Just as you wouldn't invest much effort in fixing up a rented house, our body and breath are transient and not entirely within our ownership. Our mind, on the other hand, is truly ours—free and clear. Let's ensure we give it the care and respect it deserves.

Every day, during my rounds, I encounter some or the other resident who is irritated, annoyed, or confused about their life. They grapple with questions like: Why did I join this residency? I was smart—should I have chosen engineering and gone abroad? Am I even smart enough to be here? Am I incapable of managing the work, as my senior or consultant suggests? Countless questions like these run through the minds of thousands of young residents every day.

Before starting my surgical residency at LTMMC, I spoke with a close friend and senior who was a third-year General Surgery resident there. He had known me for over 3-4 years during our MBBS. He said, "You'll learn everything you need to know as a General Surgery resident by the time you finish your residency, but be prepared for hell. There will be times when you'll break down, cry, and even consider leaving the residency and giving up on the medical field. But knowing you, I think you'll manage well."

I made it through my third year with its fair share of ups and downs, almost breaking down a few times, but I managed to keep it together. It was quite the experience! Whenever I faced a big problem, I'd ask myself: "Will this matter in the long run?" As long as the answer was "No," I stuck to my plan. I prioritized my mental health over what anyone else had to say. I never mismanaged a patient, so I didn't carry any guilt that would make me blame myself. Whatever others said or did was their problem, not mine. I knew I came to LTMMC to learn surgical skills and complete my PG, and I understood my reasons. Having a good understanding of your own feelings and abilities is absolutely essential for managing your residency. Discover yourself. You don't have to share your insecurities or problems with others, but you should definitely be aware of your insecurities, strengths, and weaknesses. And remember, a little self-awareness can save you from a lot of unnecessary drama!

Know your whys'!

When you join your residency, you will develop your skills in understanding the world. Residency is an ideal time to explore your reasons for pursuing this path. Why are you doing this residency? Why are you working so hard? By beginning to ask yourself these questions, you'll uncover many answers. Some of these answers may be uncomfortable or cause you to question yourself and your motivations. Are you driven by money? Fame? Insecurity? the prefix Dr? Or do you have a genuine interest in the field? Any of these reasons are valid. It's alright to accept your own answer, even if it is primarily about fame, family affair or money. Knowing your reasons is important, even if you don't discuss them with others or even with yourself. Like other professionals who are often judged by the salary they earn, having finances as your primary motivation should not make you feel guilty.

Nietzsche says "He who has a why to live can bear almost any how"

Thus emphasizing the importance of purpose and support in this grueling journey. After all, in the quest to heal others, residents must remember to heal themselves first.

You spend about 8-9 years learning how to manage a patient's case. But how much time have you spent learning about yourself? Now, as an adult, you're expected to handle everything—stress, anxiety, workload, sleep deprivation—often with little to no training in managing these aspects of mental health. Would you expect to ace an exam without understanding the basics? Probably not. The reason some people navigate their residency better and manage their lives more effectively, even if they haven't topped the class in the medical aspect, is that they have worked on themselves. Remember to spend time learning more about yourself. This self-discovery can improve all aspects of your life, including your interpersonal communication and stress management strategies.

> *"A person who doesn't know what the universe is, doesn't know where they are. A person who doesn't know their purpose in life doesn't know who they are or what the universe is. A person who doesn't know any one of these things doesn't know why they are here. So what to make of people who seek or avoid the praise of those who have no knowledge of where or who they are?"*
>
> **–Marcus Aurelius, Meditations**

How often do we encounter simple questions like "Who are you?" or "What do you do?" or "Where are you from?" Often dismissing them as superficial, we may not bother with more than a cursory response. However, if pressed, many people would struggle to provide a meaningful answer. Have you taken the time to deeply understand who you are and what principles you stand for? Or are you consumed by pursuits that lack significance, influenced by the wrong ideals, or following paths that leave you unfulfilled? While these questions may seem philosophical, they are crucial for self-reflection. Only by gaining clarity about yourself can you effectively navigate and manage your life and its challenges.

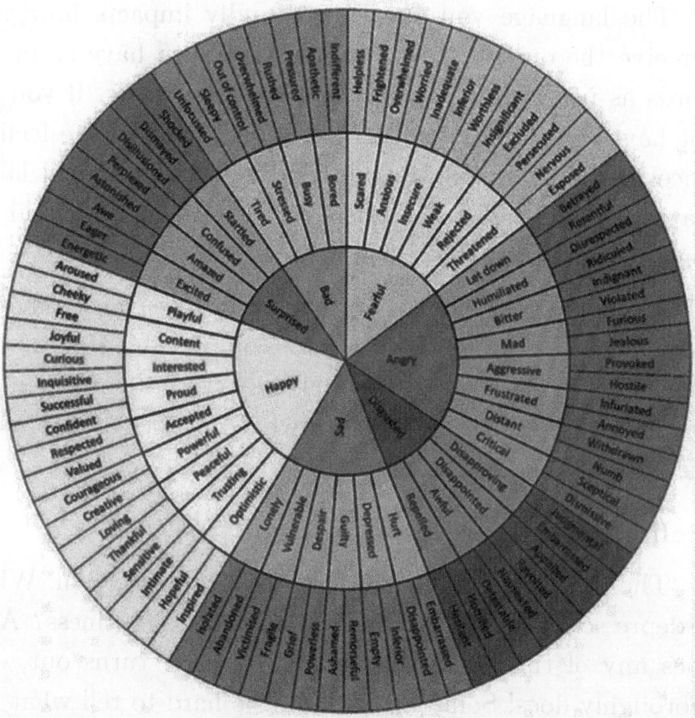

Use the feeling wheel (Wilcox, 1982) to help you find the words to describe how you feel.

What I learned from my therapist to was to ask myself, Alhad how are you feeling today? Allowing me to answer about my feelings.

The language you speak profoundly impacts how you perceive the outside world. It is essential to have as many words as possible to express how you are feeling. If you do not have the words, you can use something like the feeling wheel to give you prompts. At times, one emotional label may not be enough to encapsulate your feeling. It could be combination of feelings–I feel nervous and also excited.

Some words for emotions have progressively come to mean various things, leading to complexity. Happy has become an umbrella term for anything positive, to the extent that none of us really know that what qualifies as happy.

If I feel playful, am I happy?

If I feel motivated, am I happy?

The same has happened to words like depression. What is depressed mood - Sadness? Numbness? Emptiness? And does any of this really matter? Well, as it turns out, out thoroughly does! Sometimes, it can be hard to tell what we are thinking and what we are feeling. We often fool ourselves into believing that we feel something (and therefore it is difficult to change) when in actuality it is a thought.

Now that you've been introduced to the emotional wheel, let's test your understanding of the difference between thoughts and feelings. For each item below, identify whether it is a thought or a feeling.

For example:

1. I feel anxious.
2. I feel that something awful will happen today.

As we get better at describing our feelings, we also improve how we approach problems. Emotions are not always simply sad or happy.

Mental Health Issues Among Medical Residents

1. *Stress and Burnout*
2. *Depression and Anxiety*
3. *Substance abuse, sleep disorders, and emotional exhaustion.*

My OPD as a psychologist in a Municipal Hospital begins at dot 09:00 am, it's raining cats and dogs, my umbrella barely cooperating and the kaal-peeli outwardly rejecting to take me to the hospital – PHEW! I am half drenched and how would I go like this to the OPD as I am the Head Clinical Psychologist. What will people say? How can I go so shabby? What if I am judged? My JR & SR's who look upto me would think how beautifully I give lectures on time management and here I am all messed up.

What do I do in my practice? Take a break and process these questions:

1. What am I feeling right now?
2. Are you sure of the feeling you are feeling?
3. What is contributing to my current mood?
4. What is my go-to responses?

Everyone feels low or down from time to time. It does not always mean something is wrong or a psychological concern. Feeling low is common after distressing events or major life changes, but sometimes periods of low mood happen for no obvious reason and doesn't always mean there is something wrong with you.

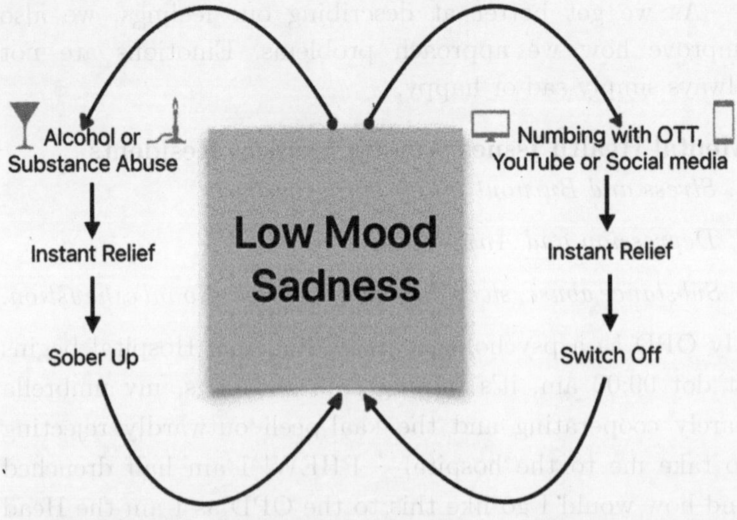

The vicious cycle of instant relief (Adapted from the work of Isabel Clark; 2017)

In Zen, they speak of 'Walking hand-in-hand'

This means going through life with those in whom we truly believe and trust – including our essential selves. The things that enable us to safeguard our memories are in no small part responsible for this feeling as well.

A. Resident Burnout

Medical residency is characterized by intense work schedules, high-stakes responsibilities, and significant emotional, physical stress and always on the go!

Defining Stress and Burnout

I define stress as a state where my decision-making skills are impaired, leading to poor problem solving, and leaving me feeling perpetually overwhelmed. When we mention stress, we often associate it negatively, thinking of it as an undesirable state. However, we all need stress in our lives! Why? The term "stress" is frequently misused. The more accurate terms are probably "distress" and "eustress."

Distress: Distress is the negative form of stress that can have detrimental effects on one's physical and mental health. It arises when demands exceed an individual's coping abilities, leading to feelings of helplessness, anxiety, and fatigue.

Eustress: Eustress, on the other hand, is the positive form of stress that can be beneficial and motivating. It occurs when stressors are perceived as challenges that can be overcome, leading to personal growth and enhanced performance. Eustress can result from positive life events such as starting a new job, getting married, or pursuing a challenging goal. It is what carried you through the challenging badminton match or allowed you to do an emergency laparotomy or an emergency C-Section.

"Burnout is what happens when you try to avoid being human for too long."

Burnout & Bandages

In the land of scrubs and latex gloves,
Where caffeine flows and no one shoves,
There's a tale, both bleak and amusing,
Of residents who long for more funding.

With bleary eyes and sagging feet,
They race the clock and skip their sleep,
Yet somewhere in the midnight hour,
They dream of life with more than power.

Code blues and rounds, they navigate,
With brains half-mushed and hearts sedate,
They pray for lunch that isn't chips,
And fantasize of long-lost trips.

"Oh joy!" they say, "another night!
Another chance to feel just right,
To learn the art of counting sheep,
While suturing a wound so deep."

Their mentors preach, "You're almost there!"
As if that soothes the thousand-yard stare,
They laugh to keep from shedding tears,
And count down days, not just the years.

Burnout & Bandages

Through chaos, mess, and patients' snore,
They find the strength to heal some more,
For though they're tired and sleep-deprived,
Their humor keeps their hope alive.

So cheers to those who laugh and mend,
With hearts so big, they never bend,
In the halls of relentless labor,
They find no time to savor its flavor.

Dr. Alhad Naragude

Burnout is a specific type of chronic work-related stress, characterized by three main components:

1. *Emotional exhaustion:* feeling drained and fatigued.

2. *Depersonalization:* developing a cynical attitude towards patients and work.

3. *Reduced personal accomplishment:* feeling ineffective and doubting one's abilities.

Burnout is particularly concerning in medical residency due to its impact on both the residents' health and patient care quality.

Prevalence of Stress and Burnout in Medical Residency

Research indicates that burnout affects a significant proportion of medical residents. Studies report prevalence rates ranging from 27% to 75%, depending on the specialty and specific circumstances.

"Residency isn't just about hard skills, but also softening your approach to yourself."

Contributing Factors

1. Workload and work hours

I still remember my average sleep being around 4 hours throughout my 1st year and had improved to 5 hours in 2nd & 3rd year. Medical residents in India typically work long hours, often exceeding 100-120 hours per week. Their demanding schedules include overnight shifts, weekend duties, and on-call responsibilities, leading to sleep deprivation and chronic fatigue.

2. Emotional and physical demands

The emotional burden of patient care, particularly dealing with critically ill patients, end-of-life situations, and medical errors, significantly contributes to stress. Residents often face moral dilemmas and the emotional toll of patient suffering, which can lead to emotional exhaustion and depersonalization. Moreover, the physical demands of residency, such as prolonged standing during surgeries and irregular meal times, can lead to physical exhaustion and a compromised immune system. I vividly remember listening to "Zinda" by Amit Trivedi; that song probably articulated my situation at the end of the week.

> *"Medicine is a demanding lover; sometimes you need to set boundaries to keep it from becoming an addiction."*

3. Learning environment

The educational aspect of residency, while crucial, adds another layer of stress. Residents are constantly evaluated on their performance, knowledge, and skills. The pressure to excel academically and clinically can be overwhelming, especially in a competitive environment where mistakes can have serious consequences. The hierarchical structure of medical training also contributes to stress. Residents often feel scrutinized and judged by senior physicians, which can lead to anxiety and self-doubt. The lack of positive feedback and recognition further exacerbates feelings of inadequacy and burnout.

4. Lack of autonomy

During residency, resident may have limited autonomy in decision-making, as they are still under supervision. This lack of control over their work and patient care decisions can be frustrating and demoralizing.

5. Personal life and relationships

The demanding nature of residency often leads to a poor work-life balance. Residents may struggle to find time for personal relationships, self-care, and leisure activities. The strain on personal life and the lack of social support can exacerbate feelings of stress and burnout.

Implications of Stress and Burnout

1. Impact on resident health

Burnout is associated with higher rates of depression, anxiety, substance abuse, and suicidal ideation. Chronic stress can also lead to physical health problems such as cardiovascular diseases, gastrointestinal issues, and a weakened immune response. The mental health of residents is of particular concern. The stigma associated with seeking mental health treatment within the medical profession further complicates this issue, leading many residents to suffer in silence.

2. Impact on patient care

Burnout can impair cognitive function, attention, and decision-making skills, leading to medical errors and compromised patient safety.

3. Professional consequences

Burnout leads to decreased job satisfaction, lower professional commitment, and higher turnover rates. Residents experiencing burnout are more likely to consider leaving the profession, contributing to workforce shortages. I still remember reminding myself why I had joined my residency whenever I was exhausted. The loss of experienced and skilled residents will disrupt the continuity of care and impact the overall efficiency of healthcare delivery. A single day resident strike in a government hospital can bring the entire healthcare system of that particular location to standstill!

Strategies for Mitigation

1. Institutional support/resident organisation support

Hospitals and residency programs play a crucial role in addressing stress and burnout. Institutions should prioritize creating a supportive work environment with adequate resources, including access to mental health services, wellness programs, and mentoring systems. Policies that promote work-hour limitations and ensure adequate rest periods are essential.

Well that's well written right? How much of it will happen in reality? Probably very little. The answer to this could be local resident bodies, who should promote support to new residents and teach them effective ways to manage their 1st year JRship. If you feel the burnout, visit your hospital's Psychiatry department, meet a clinical psychologist at your hospital; let them assess you.

2. Personal coping mechanisms/rituals

Encourage yourself to develop effective coping strategies is vital. This includes stress management techniques such as ***mindfulness, exercise, and adequate sleep***. You are with yourself throughout your life. Develop new habits, identify how you cope with stress and try to develop better coping mechanisms. I remember listening to my favourite music and going for workout. Getting out of the hospital for a short 10-15 mins stroll also does wonders. Sometimes you just need to change the environment! I remember calling myself a civilian every time I went for a movie! It allowed me to remind myself that there are other things is my life that I could do to allow myself to unwind from the hospital.

And if you're overwhelmed to understand what to do, just scan the following and do as the video says.

After three months of settling into my residency, I developed a much-needed saturday ritual. Our unit's elective OT would wrap up around 2-3 pm, and I'd dash to the canteen for lunch like it was a five-star meal. Post-lunch, I'd treat myself to a men's salon visit for a glorious 30-minute session where the barber would trim my beard and give me a head massage with Navratna hair oil. Those head massages were so good, they almost made up for the six days of chaos. Back at the hospital, I'd finally take my first bath of the week, change clothes, and then take rounds. My registrar was in on the secret and, knowing how essential this ritual was after six days of relentless work, he wouldn't call me during those precious two hours.

Fast forward to my second post, around six months into the first year, most of us had lost all sensation in our feet from standing too long, walking endless steps, and getting no rest. With our efficiency levels up, my co-JR and I would sneak off for foot massages at O'Hair in Matunga. Over time, we crafted several such rituals to sneak in some much-needed relaxation amidst the madness.

"If you get tired, learn to rest, not to quit."

3. Peer support

Fostering a sense of community and peer support can mitigate feelings of isolation and loneliness. Peer support groups and debriefing sessions can allow you to share your experiences, provide mutual support, and develop coping strategies collectively. A non formal way is to sit together and have a session where you and your friends share your frustrations and learn to have empathy towards each other Or have a "bitching session". Peer support programs can be formalized within residency programs, creating structured opportunities for everyone to connect and support one another.

In my third year, after a particularly challenging day at the hospital, I found myself struggling to manage a situation that seemed beyond my control. I reached out to my former registrar, who had been my JR3 when I was a JR1, and asked for his advice. He guided me through the situation with examples of how I could navigate it effectively. Did I handle it well? No. However, talking to my former registrar reduced my anxiety about the situation since he had faced scenarios that are far more challenging. It all boiled down to understanding that some things are not within my control. I can't change how someone else feels and reacts to a situation. I was worried about the hierarchy's backlash, where anything and everything was often blamed on the registrar. I had minimal to no contribution to the chaos. A few wise words from my former registrar helped me reach an emotional equilibrium. I learned that I can't change how someone else reacts. Our seniors have faced problems similar to ours, so it's important to ask for help.

"Don't be ashamed of needing help. You have a duty to fulfill just like a soldier on the wall of battle. So what if you are injured and can't climb up without another soldier's help?"

–Marcus Aurelius in Meditations

No one ever said you were born with all the tools you'd need to solve every problem you'd face in life. In fact, as a newborn you were actually helpless. Someone helped you then, and you came to understand that you could ask for that help. It was how you knew you were loved. Well, you are still loved. You can ask anyone for help. You don't have to face everything on your own. If you need help, comrade, just ask!!

4. Education and awareness

Training programs should include psycho-education on recognizing and addressing burnout, as well as promoting a culture that encourages seeking help without stigma. The glorification of overwork, grueling schedules, sleep deprivation, immense pressure to perform, and relentless demands are often seen as a badge of honor in residency. However, awareness begins with recognizing that your own health matters too. Strive to be a supportive senior when you reach your 2nd or 3rd year of residency. Ensure your junior has had food and stand up for them if they struggle to negotiate with paramedics or nurses. If necessary, advocate for them in conflicts with ward boys or sisters. Demonstrating that you are a team and that they are not alone can make a significant difference. Supporting each other fosters a healthier and more collaborative environment, ultimately benefiting everyone involved.

"It's not the load that breaks you down, it's the way you carry it."

5. Flexible work arrangements

Implementing flexible work arrangements, such as part-time schedules or sabbatical options, can help residents manage their workload and personal commitments more effectively. Providing options for career breaks or reduced hours during particularly challenging periods can prevent burnout. Flexible scheduling can allow residents to have more control over their work-life balance, reducing the risk of burnout.

I had an alternate Sunday off from all duties during 1st year of my residency in Urology. Me and my co-JR would manage the entire ward and ER work alone for alternate Sundays, allowing the other to rest and recover. I remember going out for lazy morning breakfast, sleeping in afternoon and again going out for some movie or dinner with friends. That Sunday would mean everything for us. We would ensure that we did our job well so the other gets to rest. Even today as a senior I understand the importance of that Sunday for my junior. We as seniors now make sure we adjust our Sundays according to the junior's schedule! Remember when you become a senior to allow your juniors the opportunity to relax and learn at the same.

B. Substance (AB)Use

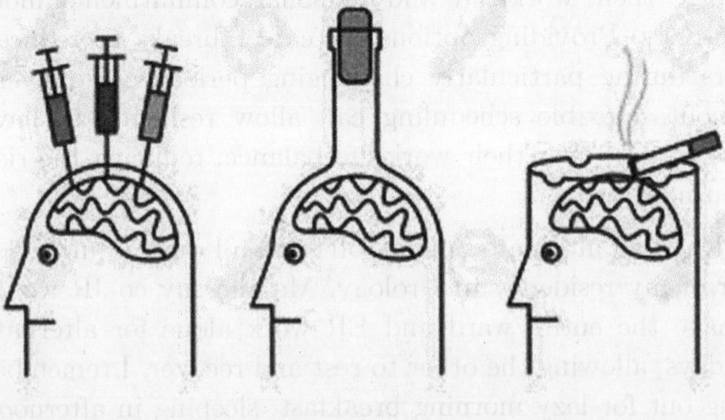

Substance (ab)use among medical professionals, particularly those in residency, is a critical issue that has far-reaching implications for individual health, patient care, and the healthcare system as a whole. Medical residency is a transition where you have money to spend, less time for yourself and probably ample access to substances.

Prevalence of Substance Abuse in Medical Residency
A study published in JAMA in 2012 revealed that approximately 10-15% of physicians will have a substance use disorder at some point during their careers, with many starting during residency. Commonly abused substances include alcohol, benzodiazepines, stimulants, and opioids.

Most of us know that residency has a way of pushing us to try everything. Escapes from ward duties and late-night parties become part of the residency culture. And why not? After a grueling week of work, I still remember those wild saturday nights. It was our escape from the hospital grind. We needed that pressure cooker to blow off steam.

Crossroads of Coping

"In the midst of charts and patient care,
Where time is scarce and stress lays bare,
A whisper lingers, a tempting snare,
As thoughts drift to a place less rare.

Marijuana's haze, a gentle sigh,
To ease the mind and pacify,
Amid the chaos, it draws them near,
A fleeting comfort, a silent cheer.

But smoking's grip, a burning hold,
Leaves lungs to ache, and hearts grow cold.
In nicotine's embrace they find,
A moment's peace, a clouded mind.

And alcohol, with its deceptive charm,
Offers solace from the day's alarm,
A toast to trials they can't ignore,
In spirits strong, they crave for more.

Yet amidst the haze, they pause to see,
The toll it takes on clarity,
For in the journey, they must find,
A balance true, a healing kind.

Crossroads of Coping

In medical residency's relentless race,
They seek resilience, find their place,
For patient care and self-care too,
They navigate the foggy view.

In the quest to heal and mend,
Let wisdom steer, let hearts defend,
Against the temptations' subtle sway,
In dedication, find the true pathway."

Dr. Alhad Naragude

But here's the thing: while the occasional escape is sometimes needed, if it becomes a habit, it's a slippery slope. Most of us at those parties danced, had a drink, and some smoked. A few took it too far. Suddenly, smoking 1-2 packs of cigarettes a day became the new normal. Others needed a 90 ml nightcap to get by.

Youth and residency are times of exploration, where individuals are particularly susceptible to the allure of instant gratification. The search for identity, the craving for acceptance, and the desire to escape pain can drive young minds toward substances that promise quick relief or euphoria. Philosophically, it is like trying to fill an existential void with a leaky bucket.

When traditional sources of meaning—like family, community, and purposeful activity—fail to provide a sense of purpose, substances step in as a tempting but deceptive alternative. They offer an illusion of control and escape, like putting a Band-Aid on a bullet wound. Instead of addressing the real issues, they just cover them up with a temporary fix, leaving the deeper problems unresolved.

At first, you're curious about the substance and start exploring it. If you enjoy it, it can turn into a habit, which may lead to dependency and eventually addiction.

> ***"The pressure of residency can drive even the strongest to seek an escape. Remember, a temporary high is not worth a permanent low."***

Remember, a little fun can be a great stress reliever, but don't let it become another round-the-clock duty! Know your limits; moderation and setting boundaries can help make better decisions and keep things in control.

Once you're addicted, you might start defending its use by convincing yourself that it makes you more creative, it calms your nerves, or it helps you focus better on work.

Causes of Substance Abuse in Medical Residency

Several factors contribute to the high rates of substance abuse among medical residents:

1. Stress and burnout

2. Access to medications

3. Cultural and environmental factors: The medical profession often has a culture where seeking help is viewed as a sign of weakness.

4. Mental health issues: Medical residents are at a high risk for mental health disorders such as depression and anxiety.

5. Lack of support systems: Many residents are far from their families and traditional support systems.

> *"Trying to numb the pain only makes it worse in the long run. Facing it head-on takes real courage."*

Consequences of Substance Abuse in Medical Residency

1. Impaired judgment and performance

2. Health risks: Substance abuse poses severe health risks, including the potential for overdose, development of chronic health conditions, and mental health deterioration. I recall an incident where a colleague was admitted to the ICU after consuming too much alcohol. Intubated in the ICU, he survived thanks to the hospital's prompt treatment. Another senior colleague developed acute pancreatitis and atrial fibrillation due to chronic alcohol consumption.

3. Professional repercussions: Substance abuse can lead to disciplinary actions, loss of medical licensure, and legal consequences. The stigma associated with substance use disorders can also damage a resident's professional reputation and career prospects.

4. Financial strain: The costs associated with obtaining substances, legal fees, and potential loss of employment can lead to significant financial strain for residents.

5. Interpersonal issues: Substance abuse can strain personal relationships, leading to social isolation, marital problems, and difficulties in maintaining a healthy work-life balance.

> ***"Being a resident is like being a teabag; you don't know how strong you are until you're in hot water." And sometimes, you just need a proper cup of tea, not a cocktail!***

Addressing Substance Abuse in Medical Residency

Prevention: (Resident Organisations At Institutional level should ask for these changes)

Policy Implementation: Developing and enforcing policies that limit working hours, provide adequate rest periods, and ensure a safe working environment.

Early Detection

1. Regular screening: Implementing regular screening programs for substance use can help detect issues early.

2. Peer support programs: Establishing peer support programs where residents can share their experiences and support each other.

3. Mentorship programs: Mentorship programs can provide residents with guidance and support from experienced professionals who can help identify early signs of substance use and provide appropriate advice.

Intervention

1. Confidential reporting systems: Creating confidential reporting systems where residents can report their concerns about substance use without fear of retribution can facilitate early intervention.

2. Employee assistance programs: They can provide confidential counseling and support services for residents dealing with substance use issues.

3. Rehabilitation programs: Institutions should have partnerships with rehabilitation programs that specialize in treating healthcare professionals. Institutions like Alcoholic Anonymous, Narcotics Anonymous, SMART recovery India, etc.

Several institutions in US have successfully implemented programs to address substance abuse among medical residents.

1. University of Pennsylvania Health System: The University of Pennsylvania Health System has developed a comprehensive wellness program for its residents. Since its implementation, the program has seen a significant reduction in reported substance use.

2. Mayo Clinic: The Mayo Clinic has established a Resident Assistance Program (RAP) that provides confidential counseling, mental health services, and substance use treatment for residents.

3. Massachusetts General Hospital: Massachusetts General Hospital has implemented a peer support program called the Physician Health Services (PHS).

C. Overthinking

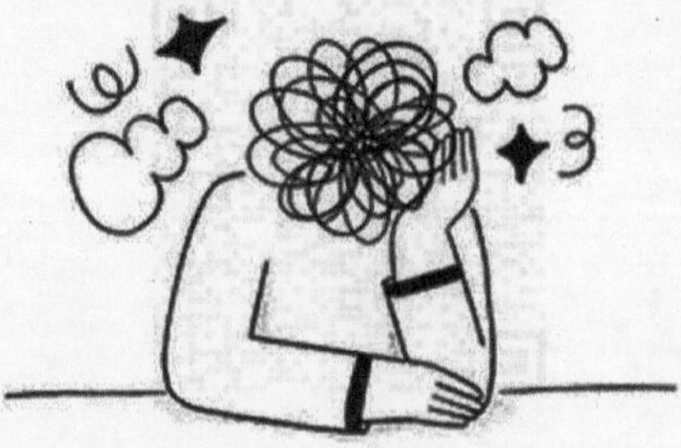

Thinking that is unhelpful and counterproductive to us is referred to as "over" thinking. Therefore, you can be excessive thinking if you find it incapable to stop thinking about the same problem while failing to come up with a solution. Despite the widely held notion that "over" thinking can be beneficial since it entails considering all relevant angles and projecting potential outcomes it yet has a positive correlation with anxiety and depressive disorders.

Take a quick tick?

- ☐ *Constantly feeling worried*
- ☐ *Unable to relax*
- ☐ *An inability to think about anything else*
- ☐ *Difficulty paying attention to work in hand*
- ☐ *Replanting the same scenario time and again*
- ☐ *Thinking of all worst-case scenarios*
- ☐ *Second guessing the decisions taken*
- ☐ *Experiencing repetitive thoughts*

Tangled in Thought

In the corridors of thought where shadows play,
Lies the snare of overthinking, leading hearts astray,
It's an endless loop, a tangled skein,
Where answers sought bring only pain.

To think too much, to spin the wheel,
Leaves the mind in knots, wounds that never heal,
For every angle viewed, and outcome dreamed,
Anxiety rises, hope dims, it seems.

Though wisdom whispers, "Consider it all,"
Excessive pondering builds a wall,
Between clarity and the endless night,
Where peace retreats from the mind's fierce fight.

In the quest for solutions, the heart is confined,
Overthinking blurs the conscious mind,
It links with shadows of despair,
Where anxious thoughts breed in the air.

So pause, dear soul, release the strain,
Let thoughts flow freely, ease the brain,
For in the balance, calm and clear,
True insight blooms, and peace draws near.

Dr. Alhad Naragude

Regardless of how many boxes have been marked, let's acknowledge that they are the result of cognitive distortions that exacerbate the symptoms of depression and anxiety. Additionally, studies have shown a high link between melancholy and overthinking (Gana et al., 2001 & Segerstrom et al., 2000).

Table of cognitive thoughts with examples

Thought Distortion	What is it?	Example
All – or – nothing thinking/ Black & white thinking	Thinking in absolutes or extremes	If I don't get the rank or seat that I am working for in my PG NEET, I am a failure!
Egocentric thinking	Assuming that others have the same perspective and values as you have and judging their behaviour through that lens	I would never be late like that. He obviously doesn't care enough about me.
Overgeneralization	Taking one event and using it to generalise about other things	I failed my exam. My future is ruined.
Musts and Shoulds	Unrealistic expectations that set us up to feel like a failure everyday	I must always look perfect. I should never do any less than my absolute best.

Challenge your negative thoughts and bust your cognitive distortions. Your thoughts are not facts! The tendency to overthink things can be decreased by learning how to reframe them in a more constructive manner.

Example:

Negative thought: My Co-JR made a mistake that had profound consequences. Why is he so stupid, now I have to redo the work.

Reframed thought: I understand mistakes can happen. I will spend extra effort to fix it. I know he is capable of doing a better job next time.

Here are some quick techniques (Japanese School of Thought) you could develop to have a better thought process and allow you to reframe your thoughts.

1. IKIGAI: To have a purpose in life. Ikigai is a Japanese concept typically translated in simple words as your *'reason for being'*. Derived from two Japanese words, 'iki' meaning life and 'kai' meaning effect, result, value, benefit, or worth, the term embodies the synthesis of a reason to live, a purpose that transcends the mundane routine of day-to-day living. It is something that drives us to get out of bed in the morning, keeps us going no matter what, and makes us feel like we're making a difference. A doctor's Ikigai might lie in helping others, instilling a sense of hope, and making a tangible difference in people's lives. Every day, she steps into the hospital, not just to perform tasks - but to contribute to the well-being of others. Ikigai can be something small or something big. In a nutshell, Ikigai is a spectrum. And the complexity of Ikigai actually reflects the complexity of life itself. Every time you feel overwhelmed remind yourself why you choose medicine. It allows you to have a broader perspective about life.

2. KAIZEN: To focus on small improvements every day and not waiting for big improvements but trying to become better by at least a percent every day.

3. SHOSHIN: To approach things with a beginner's mindset. Shoshin, a Zen Buddhist concept meaning "beginner's mind," emphasizes an attitude of openness, eagerness, and freedom from preconceptions, even when studying advanced subjects. This mindset is essential for fostering continuous learning, humility, and adaptability. Acknowledging your own weaknesses, especially when pointed out by others, can be challenging. However, approaching learning with an open mind and without preconceptions can significantly enhance your skills and patient management. I recall having to relearn certain dissection techniques during my early months in Urology residency, despite having previously mastered them during my MS. It wasn't easy, but accepting that there was a better method allowed me to adopt a beginner's perspective and improve my approach.

D. Anxiety

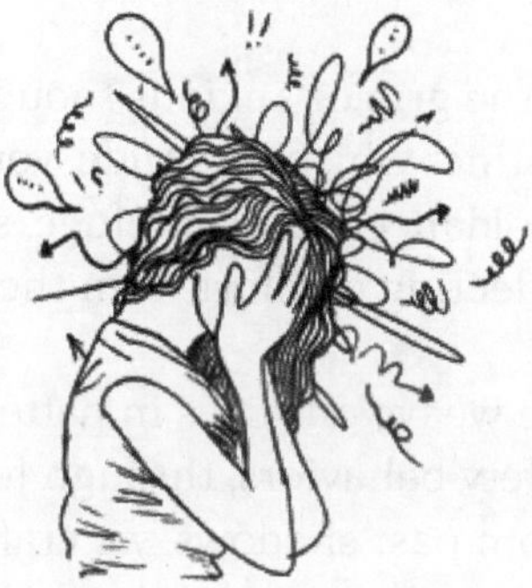

Things we do that worsen anxiety!

When we are anxious about something, the most instinctive response is to avoid it. We know that staying away will make us feel safer. We, as humans, develop safety behaviours based on what we have previously experienced to numb the anxiety we feel in the present moment. However, avoidance not only maintains anxiety but intensifies it over time.

Here's a quick overview of some safety behaviours that reduce anxiety in the moment but keeps us hooked in the long run:

1. Escape: Whether it be in the ward or during your viva, when anxiety hits you have the urge to get out of there as quickly as possible.

2. Anxious avoidance: The moment you say no to that date to avoid the anxious feeling, you are rewarded with instant feeling. Phew, I don't have to feel what I felt in my last date. But the longer you stay away from it, the fear seemingly grows.

Strength Beyond Fear

In the grip of anxious thought, we shy away,
Instinct whispers, "Hide, you'll be okay."
Avoidance seems a refuge, safe and near,
A fleeting comfort from the looming fear.

We weave our lives in patterns worn,
Safety behaviors, through fear, are born.
From past shadows, we craft a shield,
To numb the dread that won't be healed.

But hiding from the storm feeds its might,
Avoidance fans the flames, dims the light.
What seems a shelter, a quiet retreat,
Becomes a prison, a repeated beat.

For anxiety, when left unchallenged, grows,
A vine that tightens, ever close.
The more we flee, the more it calls,
Until we're bound within its walls.

So face the fear, step into the fray,
With courage drawn from each new day.
Embrace the struggle, let it be known,
That growth and peace come from the
unknown.

Strength Beyond Fear

For in the heart of every storm we see,
Lies the path to strength and serenity.
And though the journey may be long,
Facing our fears makes us strong.

Dr. Alhad Naragude

Quick Relief: Palm Technique

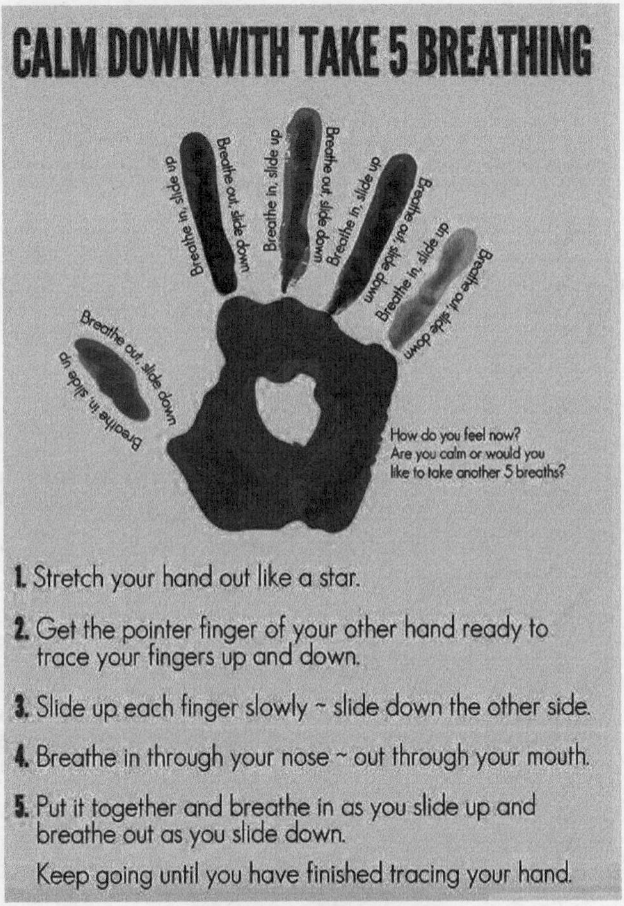

Square Breathing

This technique, known as combat or tactical breathing, is a great way to alleviate stress and relax. This breathing technique has been utilized by first responders, the military, and athletes to concentrate, establish control, and manage stress. Furthermore, it tends to aid with anxiety.

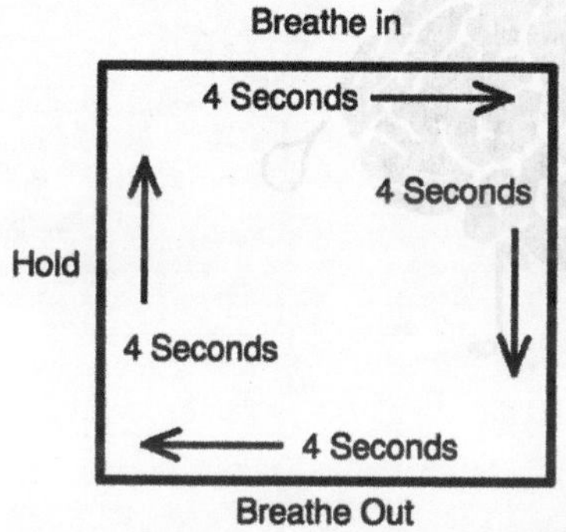

If you're struggling with anxiety and feel misunderstood, remember that our ancient brains function similarly. Anxiety is a common experience; what matters is how you manage it. Watching the movie "Inside Out" (both parts) can provide valuable insight into the workings of your brain.

Practices and Recommendations for an Overall Better Mental Health

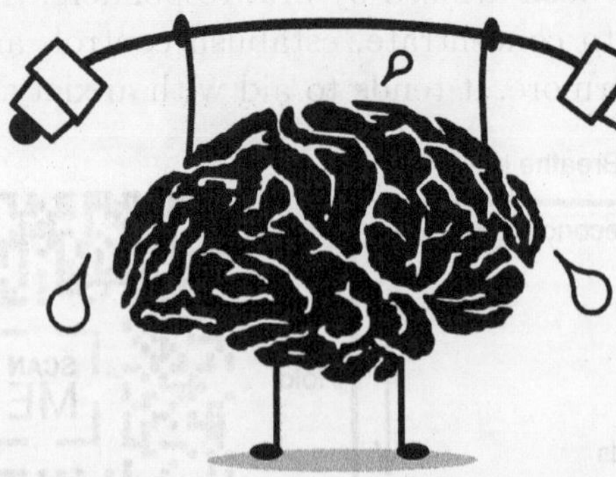

Reducing Stigma

Just like physical examination period in school, why not have a period for mental health? Many of my medical resident students tell me that they've studied psychology/psychiatry but yet don't understand what is the big deal!

Today if you are having an irritable bowel syndrome, you'll just pop a pill to feel at ease as quickly as possible but today if you're having an irritable mood which has been persistent across 7 days straight, you'll yet fight with yourself and say this too shall pass? – why such an injustice? Probably, being a medico, it's easy for you to pop a pill too, but unlike pharmacotherapy that helps alleviating symptoms, you again complain of a relapse then it's your inner core complex that needs to be fixed/attended to but where do we have the time or insight to do so?

Each of the hospitals have a Psychiatry OPD, my suggestion would be to go take a quick consult with the Clinical Psychologist in there – take a few assessments to verify what happening with you, I am sure of them navigating you further and you'll could mutually decide the further course of action.

"We all have Stress in our lives; That's to be expected!"

During the first few months of my student's post-doc at a hospital, Akash Mehta, PhD, felt overwhelmed by his work and family responsibilities. He was constantly scrambling to find babysitters and rushing to get out of work in time to pick up his children from daycare before the daycare center closed, he was also on call evenings and weekends. Although he was able to fulfil his responsibilities at work, he was very stressed and exhausted. Midway through his post-doc year, I allowed him to reduce his work week to three-and-a-half days per week by extending his commitment from 14 months to 17 months. The extra day-and-a-half off made a huge difference for him. It allowed him to take care of all sorts of family matters and take his children to the garden thrice a week. The trade off was that he had to work a lot harder and be much more efficient on the days that he'd come to work, but clinically to me he appeared as a much happier and relaxed person. Like Akash, many of my residents today are faced with juggling a multitude of demands in their professional and personal lives. From caring for their aging parents, to managing patient deliveries that can keep them "on call" day and night, residents are discovering the challenges and the benefits of balancing work, family and other responsibilities in their lives. When hospital work and family demands conflict with each other, the negative effects may include psychological distress, physiological concerns, decreased work performance and decreased job and life satisfaction.

Incorporating Self-care Activities in Your Life

Get back to your cycling, reading, listening to music, going for an ice-cream or merely getting on top of the terrace to watch the sun set. May be upskilling your singing, going for a haircut, beard trimming, some cucumbers on the eyes and rubbing ice on your face would suffice too.

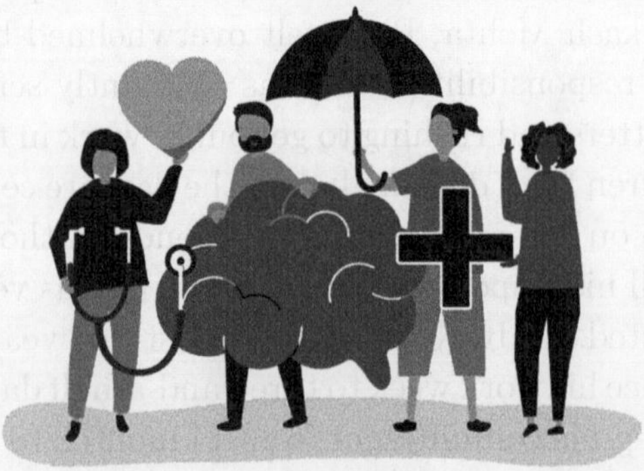

1. Develop a social support network

In the world of notifications, some notifications do make us smile. I advise my residents, especially those who are away from their homes to seek out and develop social support networks at work. In addition, informal sharing with friends and fellow colleagues and personal psychotherapy does bring some homeostasis in our functioning.

2. Don't let work take over your life

Ward rounds, on-call duties, periphery postings, research proposals, heavy OPD's, toxicity in the department, hierarchical work culture contributes to you as a resident not you as an individual. Work-life balance helps you to avoid over-identifying with one role. Identifying with multiple roles important to you makes you healthier than identifying with a single role of being a resident as long as the multiple roles are not overwhelming.

3. Embrace flexibility

Give yourself some wiggle room, will you? Come on, you have to protect your own time and make decisions right for you! Flexibility is working differently. I will work later at night after my kids are asleep, so I can spend time with them before they go to sleep. And generally, I don't schedule patients at 07:00 am.

4. Adopting a long-range perspective

Work-life balance is difficult and different for different people. You may not be able to strike the perfect balance everyday but probably can work towards having a balanced week, month or a fortnight. We all need to find steps that work for us. Don't we?

Ask Yourself a Question

If you have lingering gastrointestinal symptoms such as heartburn, indigestion, dyspepsia, bloating and constipation – how long would you wait? A week? A fortnight? A month? No! right? You're a resident doctor, you know the medicine, you'll read and manage it right? And if you fail at managing the symptoms you'll probably show to someone.

Then why such an unequal treatment with your persisting negative thoughts, irrational beliefs, fears, low mood, gender dysphoria etc.? We stretch, flex and sometimes even pray for all our thinking to magically go away. Self-talk like, this too shall pass; I am stronger that I think can help but they still remain.

We also tell ourselves, "Let's take professional help." But this specific thought is like a boomerang, we keep going back and forth failing multiple times to take execute our decision. When your mental health fluctuates, it can be even more difficult to make decisions and take action. So seeking the help you need becomes harder to do. And, there is no set of rules that tells you when to see a professional. Many of us also believe that we don't deserve it because we internally compare ourselves with our co-JR's and their little history we know which we think it's worse and if they can sail through these big waves so can I! By that time, the hill to climb has become a mountain. Waiting until your deathbed before seeking help is never a good strategy for maintaining your health, both mentally and physically. In an ideal world, therapy should be available to everyone, if not just being there for one another and having the human connect helps too. We must remember that mental health is simply an aspect of one's overall physical health. Let's continue to help each other by talking openly and honestly about mental health and doing everything we can to normalize mental health and eliminate stigma.

Until we start to view mental illness as an illness that impacts your brain the same way we view an illness that affects your heart or your kidneys, we'll continue to face the devastating consequences caused by stigma.

References:

1. Roberta L. Nutt, PhD, chair of the APA Board of Professional Affairs' Advisory Committee on Colleague Assistance (ACCA), American Psychological Association.
2. Jamison, D., & O'Mara, J. (1991). Managing workforce 2000. San Francisco: Jossey-Bass.
3. Pope, K.S., & Vasquez, M.J.T. (2005). How to survive and thrive as a therapist: Information, ideas, and resources for psychologists. Washington, DC: American Psychological Association.
4. Quick, J.C., & Tetrick, L.D. (Eds.). (2002). Handbook of Occupational Health Psychology.
5. Scandura, T.A., & Lankau, M.J. (1997). Relationships of gender, family responsibility, and flexible work hours to organizational commitment and job satisfaction.
6. Stamm, B.H. (1999). Secondary traumatic stress: Self-care issues for clinicians, researchers, and educators. (2nd ed.). Baltimore: Sidran.

E. Suicide

Every month we hear about a resident's suicide. Its buzzes on the social media for a few days. People who were close to the person are affected and rest continue their routine. A topic sensitive yet crucial to address.

The cumulative effect of varied challenges in residency can significantly impact the mental health of residents and increase their vulnerability to suicide. Studies have shown that healthcare professionals, especially residents in training, have higher rates of burnout, depression, anxiety, and suicidal ideation compared to the general population.

Theoretically jargon apart what can you do to help your friends and colleagues? If you notice behavioral changes or signs that a friend or colleague may be struggling with their mental health or potentially suicidal, it's crucial to approach the situation with empathy and care. Here are some steps and questions you can consider:

Signs to Watch For:

- **Behavioral changes:** Withdrawal from social activities, changes in sleep or eating patterns, increased substance use.
- **Emotional changes:** Persistent sadness, hopelessness, or irritability.
- **Changes in self-care:** Neglecting personal hygiene, not eating or sleeping well.
- **Verbal cues:** Expressions of feeling trapped, being a burden, or having no reason to live.
- **Giving away possessions:** Making arrangements or giving away prized possessions.

Pulse of Perseverance

In the crucible of residency's fire,
Where dreams and duties both aspire,
Days blend into endless toil,
Testing resolve and inner soil.

Amongst the pressures that abound,
A doctor's soul can be profound.
Yet in the struggle, don't lose sight,
Of the passion that ignites the fight.

Each patient's story, each battle won,
Speaks of courage beneath the sun.
Hold fast to hope, let compassion lead,
In every moment of human need.

For in the unity of those who care,
Lies the strength to rise and dare.
Through every hardship, stand with pride,
Knowing resilience walks beside.

In the journey's length and breadth,
Find solace, even in the depth.
For in this noble path you tread,
Remember, you're not alone ahead.

Dr. Alhad Naragude

Questions to Ask to Assess Suicide Risk:

- Have you been feeling more down or hopeless than usual?
- Do you find yourself thinking that things would be better if you weren't here?
- Have you thought about hurting yourself or ending your life?
- Have you made any plans or taken any steps towards hurting yourself?
- Do you have access to means (like pills or weapons) that you could use to harm yourself?
- Have you been drinking more alcohol or using drugs more than usual?

Interventions

Intervening when you suspect someone may be at risk of suicide requires sensitivity, compassion, and prompt action. Here are steps you can take to intervene effectively:

1. Initiate a conversation

Approach the person in a private and non-judgmental setting. Express your concern for their well-being and mention specific observations that have raised your concern. If you know the person well, chances are they will express themselves to you.

2. Ask directly about suicide

Be direct but compassionate in your approach. Ask questions such as:

- "Are you thinking about hurting yourself?"
- "Have you thought about committing suicide?"
- Asking directly can help clarify the person's intentions and open the door for them to talk about their feelings.

3. Listen actively

Allow the person to express their feelings without interrupting or judging. Validate their emotions and let them know you are there to support them.

4. Offer support

Encourage them to seek help from a mental health professional or counselor. Offer to accompany them to an appointment or help them find resources, such as crisis hotlines or support groups.

5. Remove access to means

If possible, remove any objects or substances that could be used for self-harm. This may include medications, firearms, or other potentially harmful items.

6. Stay connected and follow up

Follow up with the person regularly to check on their well-being. Show that you care and are available to listen and support them through difficult times.

7. Involve trusted individuals

Encourage the person to reach out to friends, family members, or other supportive individuals. In some cases, involving a trusted person in their support network can provide additional resources and perspectives.

8. Seek professional help

If the person is in immediate danger or you are unsure how to proceed, seek assistance from a mental health professional, crisis intervention team, or emergency services. Do not hesitate to call emergency services if you believe the person is at imminent risk of harm.

Suicide Helpline Numbers

Hold On

In the quiet depths where shadows roam,
A heart in turmoil finds no home.
Yet in the darkness, a glimmer may start,
A whispered hope within the heart.

Hold on, dear soul, through the night's
embrace,
For dawn will come with gentle grace.
In every ache and tear you cry,
Know you're not alone—please, don't say
goodbye.

Dr. Alhad Naragude

Chapter 6

RELATIONSHIPS

For believers in the power of love to overcome all obstacles, it's heartening to discover that love can triumph even in the face of the daunting challenges of residency. Amidst 3 years of rigorous medical education, single medical students often find themselves preoccupied with more than just memorizing drugs and bugs. Indeed, the hallowed halls of medical school have been witness to countless love stories, where the sparks of romance ignite and lasting bonds are forged. Love knows no bounds of time or circumstance, and it can strike unexpectedly, weaving its magic into the lives of student couples who embark on their journey together.

Today, it's a common sight to see graduating classes filled with student couples, their love stories intertwined with the pursuit of medical knowledge and professional growth. These couples courageously navigate the trials of residency hand in hand, their commitment to each other unwavering despite the distance and demands of their respective training programs. Some are fortunate enough to secure positions in the same city, reveling in the joy of shared experiences and cherished moments together. Yet, for others, fate may decree a path of separation, as they find themselves in different cities, bound by the thread of a long-distance relationship that tests the strength of their love and devotion.

Amidst the hustle and bustle of hospital corridors and late-night study sessions, love blossoms, defying the odds and illuminating the darkest of days with its radiant glow. For those who dare to believe, love conquers all, casting its enchanting spell over the tumultuous journey of residency and beyond.

The demanding nature of medical residency can strain relationships in various ways, affecting both romantic partnerships and family dynamics.

Hearts and Histology

In halls where medical students are fraught,
With bugs, drugs, and thoughts
overwrought,
Two hearts sneak in some romance flair,
Amidst anatomy and stethoscope wear.

Between lectures and all-nighters grim,
Love sneaks in on a whim,
A spark amidst the histo-slides,
Love can't be bound by class divides.

Between "Name that rash" and "Suture this
cut,"
A wink, a smile, "You're the balm to my rut."
Love's embrace will never stray,
Through the hustle, come what may.

So while diagnosing a tricky rash,
Remember love can make a splash,
In residency's chaos, love still finds,
A way to mend two frantic minds.

Dr. Alhad Naragude

1. Time Constraints: Long work hours and unpredictable schedules leave residents with limited time for personal pursuits, including spending quality time with their partners and families.

Feelings of Neglect: One of the primary consequences of time constraints during residency is the feeling of neglect experienced by partners and family members. When residents are constantly immersed in their work, their loved ones may feel overlooked or undervalued, leading to resentment and hurt feelings. Partners may perceive the long hours and frequent absences as prioritizing work over the relationship, causing emotional strain and discord. Partners may become frustrated with the constant interruptions to plans and the inability to make long-term commitments due to the unpredictable nature of residency schedules. Residents, in turn, may feel resentful of the sacrifices they must make in their personal lives to meet the demands of their medical training. Conversations where your partner expresses sentiments like "It feels like we hardly see each other anymore" or "We haven't had a proper meal together in days" can evoke a deep sense of sadness and longing. It's overwhelming to manage a list of missed calls from old friends and family members, reminding you of the countless gatherings and events you've missed. The weight of missing weddings, family vacations, and numerous lunches and dinners with loved ones weighs heavily on your heart. I vividly recall missing out on so many weddings, including those of my closest friends, where I couldn't even attend a single day of their celebrations. It's a painful memory that lingers, highlighting the sacrifices made during the demanding journey of residency. Family members would often find me sleeping on off days or leave from work. The only time I went home during my residency was when I had fever! Most of my colleagues either had dengue or COVID when their leaves were approved!

2. Emotional Exhaustion: Emotional exhaustion manifests as a heavy burden that seeps into personal relationships, leading residents to become irritable, emotionally distant, or prone to mood swings. My married friend would return home after a grueling 36-hour shift would find himself snapping at his wife over trivial matters, unable to muster the patience or emotional capacity for meaningful communication. The emotional toll of witnessing suffering and loss in the hospital would leave many residents feeling numb and withdrawn, making it challenging to engage in intimate and empathetic interactions with even their loved ones.

3. Physical Exhaustion: Chronic fatigue! A syndrome many of my colleagues believed they suffered from. After completing back-to-back shifts in the hospital, many returned home too exhausted to engage in physical activities or intimate moments with their partner. The long hours spent on their feet, attending to patients' needs, would leave them physically depleted, with little energy left to invest in their relationships. This diminished capacity for physical affection and intimacy had strained the connection between them and their partners, as well as impacted their ability to fully participate in shared activities or outings with loved ones. Normal activities such as shopping or going out to movies were replaced by swigging dinner and watching Netflix. No outings for months!

4. Financial Strain: Entering residency, typically between the ages of 24 to 30, is a pivotal stage where individuals grapple with their own unique financial challenges that can deeply affect relationships. The modest salaries offered to residents, ranging from 40,000 to 1,10,000 in India, often ignite feelings of pressure. Take, for instance, a resident who feels the weight of guilt for not contributing equally to shared expenses like rent or household bills due to their limited income. This burden of guilt can sow seeds of tension and resentment in the relationship, as the partner may feel overwhelmed by the financial responsibilities they bear alone. Furthermore, the limitations imposed by residency salaries can deeply impact the couple's lifestyle, stripping away the joy of shared leisure activities. Picture a scenario where they must reluctantly forego vacations, dining out, or other simple pleasures due to tight budgets. A single room-kitchen would have rent of around 35,000 to 40,000 in and around hospitals in Mumbai! Thats half the salary paid only on rent. This deprivation could dim the spark of excitement in many relationships & also stifles the ability to create cherished memories together. It casts a long shadow over future aspirations and planning within the relationship. Consider the weighty decision to delay significant life milestones like buying a home or starting a family due to financial insecurity. Adding to the emotional burden is the responsibility many residents carry to support their families financially. Any delay in achieving stability can exacerbate the sense of unease and anxiety within family dynamics, as the pressure to provide looms heavy over their heads. A few of my colleagues would send some fixed amount of their salaries to home.

5. Role Changes: Transitioning from medical school to residency marks a profound shift in roles, both professionally and personally, with unique challenges in the Indian context. Residents often grapple with balancing their identity as a physician with their roles as partners, parents, or children, which can ignite conflicts and identity crises within relationships. For instance, a resident may find themselves torn between the demands of their rigorous training and the expectations of their traditional Indian family. The pressure to excel in their medical career while fulfilling familial duties can create a sense of guilt and internal conflict, straining relationships as they navigate conflicting priorities.

Residents may struggle with asserting their autonomy and authority at work, only to come home to familial expectations of obedience and deference. This juxtaposition of roles can lead to feelings of inadequacy and frustration, as residents grapple with reconciling their professional and personal identities.

Furthermore, cultural expectations regarding marriage and family life in India can add another layer of complexity to the transition to residency. Married residents may face pressure to balance their professional ambitions with their spouse's career aspirations, navigating societal norms around gender roles and household responsibilities. This balancing act can strain marital relationships, leading to conflicts over division of labor, time management, and decision-making.

6. Isolation and Loneliness: The hierarchical structure of medical institutions often fosters a competitive and isolating environment, where many feel reluctant to reach out for support or camaraderie from their peers. The emphasis on hierarchy and authority could hinder the development of meaningful social connections within the workplace, leaving them feeling isolated and disconnected. Moreover, the cultural stigma surrounding mental health issues in India, further exacerbate feelings of isolation. The fear of being perceived as weak or incompetent prevents residents from seeking help or opening up about their struggles with loneliness and isolation which leads to a cycle of silence and internalized distress. Because *log kya kahengay* matters more to us!

The demanding nature of schedules leaves little time to nurture social connections outside of work. Long hours, overnight shifts, and weekend duties consume the majority of their time and energy, making it challenging to maintain friendships, attend social gatherings, or participate in community activities. What options are left to socialise? Tinder, Bumble! Swiping right and left to make new connections.

7. Mismatched Priorities: Women in residency face unique challenges when it comes to mismatched priorities between career advancement and family obligations.

Many women in India still bear the primary responsibility for household chores and caregiving duties, even while pursuing their medical careers. This dual burden often results in a conflict between the time and energy required for professional development during residency and the expectations of providing emotional support and stability within the family. As a result, female residents may experience resentment and friction within their relationships as they struggle to balance their career aspirations with their familial responsibilities. Moreover, societal expectations regarding marriage and motherhood further exacerbates the mismatched priorities for women in residency. Pressure to marry at a young age and start a family can clash with the demands of a rigorous residency schedule, leading to conflicts between personal desires and professional ambitions. They may find themselves torn between the desire to advance in their medical careers and the expectation to prioritize family life, resulting in tension and resentment within their relationships.

Additionally, the lack of support systems and workplace policies tailored to the needs of women in residency is can compound these challenges. Women may face difficulties accessing childcare services or maternity leave benefits, further hindering their ability to balance work and family responsibilities.

Strategies

Despite the significant challenges posed during residency, there are strategies that most residents and their partners can employ to navigate these difficulties and maintain a healthy relationship:

1. Open communication: Honest and transparent communication is indeed crucial for navigating the impact of time constraints on relationships, but its effectiveness may vary depending on individual circumstances. While open dialogue can lay the foundation for understanding and compromise, it often requires considerable effort and time for both partners to reach a place of effective communication. For instance, consider a scenario where a resident consistently communicates their struggles with time constraints to their partner, expressing the need for understanding and support. Despite these efforts, the partner may struggle to fully grasp the extent of the resident's challenges at times despite being a medical resident themselves! or may inadvertently minimize their concerns, leading to frustration and tension in the relationship.

Similarly, cultural or societal factors may hinder effective communication between partners, particularly in the Indian context. For example, traditional gender roles and expectations may discourage open expression of emotions or vulnerabilities, making it difficult for residents and their partners to have honest conversations about the impact of time constraints on their relationship.

Men may find sharing their emotions particularly challenging! I will be perceived as weak if I tell her that I'm struggling with my work is what often goes through their minds. *Mard ko dard nahi hota.*

Past experiences or unresolved conflicts can also impede effective communication. For instance, if someone has previously attempted to communicate their needs but felt dismissed or invalidated by their partner's response, they may be hesitant to engage in further dialogue, leading to a cycle of miscommunication and resentment.

Talk! Talk! Talk! Whatever the status of your relationship- situationship, dating, friends with benefits or whatever is the buzzing term these days. Talk your feelings. You can't understand a patient's status unless you talk with them. So is your relation! By actively listening to each other's perspectives and working together to find mutually acceptable solutions, couples can overcome misunderstandings and strengthen your relationship bonds.

Communicating your struggles with your family members (especially if you're from a non-medico background) can present its own set of challenges due to differing perspectives and expectations. A friend of mine struggled convey the demanding nature of his residency schedule to his non-medical family members, who had limited understanding of the pressures and responsibilities involved in medical training. His cousins felt that he has moved out to a bigger city and has become arrogant and self involved and doesn't hang out or talk with them enough. ***Ab tu bada aadmi ban gaya!*** Little did they know how eager he was to go and spend time with them.

Cultural factors such as the emphasis on familial obligations and hierarchy can complicate communication with family members. For instance, one may feel pressured to prioritize family gatherings or celebrations over their professional commitments, leading to conflicts as they attempt to assert boundaries and advocate for their own needs.

Language barriers or generational differences in communication styles can hinder effective dialogue with family members. Misinterpretations or misunderstandings may arise as a result. *Ab tu bada ho gaya hai, ab humari baat kaha manta hai tu! Tujhsay baat karna mushkil hai! Humey mat sikha!* You can image many more such dialogues from your family members. What can you do? TALK! Express your feelings in a way your family understands. Preparing non medical family members prior to joining residency is something you should consider seriously.

2. Quality over quantity: Focusing on quality rather than quantity of time spent together. Engage in meaningful activities together which can enrich the bond, despite limited time availability of time.

Example:

1. Setting aside a specific evening each week for a date night, whether it's cooking a new recipe together, watching a movie, or exploring a new hobby.

2. Planning a weekend getaway or day trip to nearby attractions, allowing you to escape the stress of residency and create lasting memories together.

3. Making time for regular exercise or outdoor activities, such as going for a jog in the park or taking a yoga class together, to prioritize your health and well-being as a couple.

4. Participating in volunteer work or community service projects as a team, giving back to others while strengthening your bond through shared experiences.

5. Creating a shared bucket list of activities or places you want to explore together, and actively working towards ticking off items on the list whenever possible.

By intentionally carving out time for these meaningful activities, you will deepen your connection with your partner and cultivate a sense of adventure and joy in your relationship, even amidst the demands of residency.

3. Flexibility and adaptability: Remaining flexible and adaptable is essential when managing the unpredictable nature of residency schedules. Both residents and their partners should embrace the need for spontaneity and be understanding of last-minute changes or interruptions that may arise. For instance, if a resident's shift unexpectedly extends late into the evening, instead of becoming frustrated, the couple could seize the opportunity to have a cozy dinner at home or plan a spontaneous outing once the resident returns. By embracing flexibility and creativity in their plans, the couple can make the most of their time together, despite the challenges posed by residency.

4. Prioritizing self-care: Prioritizing self-care is imperative for residents to safeguard against burnout and sustain their well-being, which in turn positively impacts their relationships. Establishing boundaries, such as setting aside dedicated time for relaxation or leisure activities, allows residents to recharge and maintain balance amidst their demanding schedules. Engaging in self-care practices such as meditation, exercise, or hobbies not only nurtures their mental and physical health but also rejuvenates their emotional connection with their partners.

5. Seeking support: Reaching out for support from friends, family members, and professional counselors can offer residents and their partners valuable emotional reinforcement during trying periods. For instance, confiding in a trusted friend about the stresses of residency or seeking guidance from a therapist.

6. 24-hour rule: My friend, Amit, who was a radiology resident, implemented a strict "24-hour rule," mandating contact from his girlfriend every day without fail. This directive ensured clarity and eliminated the uncertainty of whether his significant other would check in. For instance, whether through a phone call, a quick text saying "I miss you," or even a brief video chat, any form of acknowledgment sufficed to ease separation anxiety and maintained connection.

7. Compromise: In the whirlwind of residency, it's easy to lose sight of the blessings found in love. Appreciating the positives amidst career demands is crucial, as taking them for granted can dim the light of a full heart. By pausing to rationally consider situations that might otherwise cause offense, even in moments of stress, you can maintain balance in your relationship. Remember, neither you nor your significant other are the center of the universe. Both of you are entitled to occasional overreactions, bad days, and disagreements. While there's no perfect recipe for a relationship, insisting on an inflexible "my way or the highway" approach risks damaging harmony. Instead, prioritize compromise, allowing for healthy disagreements while aiming for mutual understanding and balance.

Long-Distance Relationships

Long-distance relationships during medical residency are a unique challenge, characterized by the demanding schedules and geographical constraints inherent in the training process. Many often find themselves separated from their partners by long distances, whether due to different residency placements, career opportunities, or educational pursuits.

One of the primary challenges of long-distance relationships in medical residency is the limited time available for communication and quality time together. Both often work long hours, including overnight shifts and weekends, leaving little opportunity for regular interaction. This can lead to feelings of loneliness, frustration, and insecurity, as both partners struggle to maintain a sense of closeness amidst the distance. Moreover, the geographical separation can also create logistical challenges, such as coordinating schedules to find time for visits. Financial constraints may also come into play, as residents may have limited resources to travel frequently or cover the expenses associated with maintaining a long-distance relationship.

Despite the hurdles, countless couples in long-distance relationships during medical residency demonstrate resilience by nurturing their bond amidst the demands of training. They harness technology's power to bridge the physical gap, engaging in heartfelt video calls, sending reassuring text messages, and sharing snippets of their lives via social media platforms. I know a friend who schedules weekly Skype dates to catch up on with his fiance. He prioritizes face-to-face interactions by planning regular visits and celebrating special occasions despite the distance. Surprise visits to his partner's place with a spontaneous weekend getaway or arranging a virtual dinner date to commemorate his anniversary.

A few of my friends broke up with their partners after separation in residency. New place, new feelings, new distractions, new people. Many found themselves lonely and started dating someone who could fill the void! Many lied to their partners or cheated. In this world of instant dating and apps to swipe right and left many found themselves in dual minds.

The foundation of successful long-distance relationships in medical residency lies in unwavering communication, trust, and empathy. Partners will need to prioritize active listening, respecting each other's schedules, and offering unwavering support during challenging times. For instance, a resident might adjust their study schedule to accommodate their partner's availability for a heartfelt conversation, demonstrating their commitment to nurturing the relationship despite the distance. Ultimately, by prioritizing each other's emotional needs, demonstrating patience and flexibility, and embracing innovative ways to maintain intimacy, couples can navigate the trials of residency together.

Breakups

Amidst the whirlwind of residency, many find themselves at a crossroads, parting ways with past loves and encountering new connections that stir their hearts. Yet, bidding farewell to a cherished relationship can unleash a torrent of emotions, leaving wounds that may take time to heal. Rather than seeking solace in the arms of another as a temporary distraction, embrace the solitude as an opportunity for introspection and self-discovery.

Navigating the aftermath of a breakup requires courage and patience, as waves of grief and longing wash over the soul. Take the time to tend to your wounded heart, allowing the echoes of past loves to fade as you journey towards inner peace and clarity. Embrace the uncertainty of the unknown, trusting that in due time, the path forward will reveal itself. Amidst the shadows of loneliness, resist the temptation to seek fleeting companionship as a means of coping. Instead, let the flickering flame of your heart guide you towards a love that is genuine and enduring.

The public nature of social media can complicate breakups. Relationship statuses, comments from friends, and even the visible absence of a partner can lead to unwanted attention and speculation. Love, breakups, and relationship labels are experienced and understood in distinct ways compared to previous generations, influenced by digital technology, social media, and evolving social norms.

Take time for yourself. You might be the most eligible bachelor or spinster in your hospital and have people lined up to date you; but take time. Flirt around, socialise, retrospect into the last relationship & understand what went wrong.

After a breakup, reflecting on the experience can help you understand yourself and the relationship better, aiding in personal growth and future relationships.

Sit down and ask yourself these questions:

1. What did I learn about myself in this relationship?
2. What were the key reasons for the breakup?
3. Were there any red flags I ignored?
4. How did I contribute to the issues in the relationship?
5. What qualities do I want in a future partner?
6. How did this relationship impact my mental and emotional health?
7. What positive aspects can I take from this experience?
8. Did I feel respected and valued throughout the relationship?
9. What can I do to heal and move forward healthily?
10. How can I improve my communication and conflict resolution skills?
11. What boundaries do I need to set for myself in future relationships?
12. How can I ensure I maintain my identity and independence in a relationship?
13. Am I ready to start dating again, or do I need more time to heal?

14. What activities or hobbies can I pursue to help rebuild my sense of self?

15. How can I better manage and express my emotions in future relationships?

16. Are you dating because you're lonely?

17. Was it just an online swiping right-left to cope with the break up?

18. Was it a rebound relationship?

19. Have I forgiven myself from the previous relationship?

Answer these questions honestly. You don't have to share the answers with anyone.

Allow your answers to change who you are. You're still young! You have room to improve yourself, build new habits. Slowly as you age it will be difficult to change habits. You'll have beliefs that are rigid and biased to your own experiences. Eventually we are just a bunch of memories and experiences. To change the way you date will need changes in yourself! Or you'll end up stuck in a pattern of dating and probably blame luck or the other sex to be the problem.

And when the time is right, when your heart is ready to love again, step forth with courage and conviction, knowing that you have stayed true to yourself. For in honoring your own desires and preferences, you pave the way for relationships that are rooted in authenticity and mutual respect. So, dare to embrace the journey of self-discovery, for it is through knowing yourself that you will find the love that you truly deserve.

"If you never heal from what hurt you, you'll bleed on someone who didn't cut you"

Renew and Reflect

Answer truly, your secrets keep,
Whispers of your soul run deep.
Let them mold and let them guide,
In youth's embrace, let change reside.

Habits harden as years advance,
Flexibility fades, a fleeting chance.
Memories, experiences, intertwine,
Defining who we are with time.

Transform yourself, break the chain,
Or in old patterns, you'll remain.
You'll be stuck in a dating rut,
Blaming bad luck or thinking the other sex
is nuts.

So take a good look, make some changes
today,
And laugh at how far you've come along the
way!

Dr. Alhad Naragude

Singlehood

For many medical residents, the intricacies of treating a patient's heart proves less daunting than navigating the quest for their own love. In India being single can carry a weighty societal stigma, where cultural norms often discourage dating before the age of 25 but exert strong pressure to marry soon thereafter. This juxtaposition leaves many young adults with limited experience in the realm of dating and relationships, struggling to find their footing in matters of the heart.

Both men and women alike encounter challenges unique to their social landscape. Some embrace their single status with contentment, finding solace and fulfillment in their independence and solitude. For them, life unfolds at their own pace, unencumbered by the responsibilities and compromises that accompany a committed relationship. Yet, amidst circles of friends who are increasingly settling into marriages or partnerships, others may find themselves grappling with feelings of loneliness or societal pressure to conform. The digital age has ushered in new avenues for seeking companionship. Many turn to online matrimonial forums or dating apps, where the swipe of a finger becomes a gateway to potential connections.

Whether you're single by choice or still searching for someone special, channel all your love towards yourself. Embrace solitude. Build resilience. Learn to fallback on yourself.

You'll have aunties asking about your relationship status and demanding laddus! "*Tu kab laddu khilayega/khilayegi?*" Learn to handle them! It's great training for dealing with unwanted questions.

If you want to be with someone, you'll have to make the effort. I still remember driving at 2 am for someone when I had barely slept for 3-4 hours. Sleep-deprived, overworked, and still putting in extra effort for someone special. It involves sacrifices. You'll probably be exhausted after a 15-16 hours workday, but you'll still need to show up! You'll watch movies you don't enjoy, make time for someone else's stories and plans. Even today, I sometimes sleep through movies in the theater! I do it because I want to.

As a single person, you can enjoy your own time. Fall in love with yourself, get comfortable in your own skin, and find peace within your mind. You'll likely attract more people once you're at peace with yourself.

LGBTQ+

Most non-heterosexual and trans-residents remain largely unknown, because open acknowledgement of homosexuality is a step taken by very few residents in the medical institutes. Nevertheless, whatever the number, many gay men and lesbian women in medicine form and maintain long-standing relationships with their partners. They too are subject to particular stresses as they do not feel comfortable being open at work about their sexual orientation or gender identity because of prejudice and discrimination against LGBTQ+, both from within and without.

Chronic shame persists, especially as we are a very culture driven society where doctors are equivalent to gods as they have the ability to protect and save lives – how can they not save themselves from same sex relationships? However, the situations are now changing and there has been a wave of retaliation and distress but fear remains!

LGBTQ+ residents are particularly vulnerable to mental health challenges, often finding themselves with no one to confide in, facing their struggles alone. In many cases, when they do reach out to faculty, they are met with ridicule and become targets of discrimination. The journey of residency is inherently isolating, with support systems—family, friends, and partners—largely cut off. This can lead to the formation of relationships between residents, driven by emotional dependency as they navigate shared hardships. These connections may stem more from attachment or habit than genuine love or affection. Additionally, the stress of residency can contribute to a hookup culture, where residents engage in relationships or make decisions that may be based more on coping with stress than true connection.

Chapter 7

PHYSICAL HEALTH AND NUTRITION

Unbalanced Care

In the grand theater of health, doctors take the stage,
Guardians of well-being, in wisdom they engage.
Advocates for lifestyles, prevention is their creed,
Yet behind white coats and stethoscopes, an irony indeed.

For many in the healing arts, neglect their own advice,
Struggling to find time for health, despite their sacrifice.
The benefits of exercise, they know within their hearts,
Yet the demands of their profession tear their wellness apart.

Sedentary ways invite a host of ills to bear,
Obesity, heart troubles, and musculoskeletal wear.
Stress and burnout follow, minds burdened and fraught,
Job satisfaction wanes, and quality of care is caught.

Patients look to doctors, their models in the fight,
But when healers neglect themselves, it undermines the light.
A doctor enters, sage advice on lips, extolling exercise,
Yet behind the scenes, laments their sedentary guise.

Unbalanced Care

Contrary to belief, their lives aren't brisk with walks,
Stethoscopes swinging, as if in endless talks.
Hunched over desks, computer screens their view,
Patients upon patients, exercise they eschew.

The rare sprint to surgery, a frantic dash through halls,
But mostly, they're seated, within their OPD walls.
Knowledge of nutrition, they hold within their grasp,
Yet succumb to comfort foods, within the stress's clasp.

From svelte to soft, the contours change with time,
Stress-eating, desk-bound lives, an unending climb.
In this irony profound, the healers need a cure,
To heed their own advice, and find a balance pure.

Dr. Alhad Naragude

The Irony of Health Guardians Neglecting Their Own Well-Being: In the grand theater of health, doctors take center stage as the guardians of well-being, tirelessly advocating for healthy lifestyle choices and disease prevention. Yet, behind the white coats and stethoscopes lies a glaring irony – many doctors themselves struggle to prioritize exercise and maintain a healthy lifestyle. In this tongue-in-cheek exploration, we delve into the curious phenomenon of doctors neglecting their own physical fitness, despite their intimate knowledge of its importance. Despite being well-versed in the benefits of exercise, many doctors struggle to prioritize physical activity due to the demands of their profession.

The consequences of this lack of exercise among doctors are manifold. Physically, sedentary behavior puts doctors at risk for a myriad of health issues, including obesity, cardiovascular disease, diabetes, and musculoskeletal problems. Mentally, the lack of physical activity can exacerbate stress, anxiety, and burnout, leading to decreased job satisfaction and lower quality of patient care. Furthermore, the example set by doctors has ripple effects throughout society. Patients look to their healthcare providers as role models for healthy living. When doctors neglect their own health, it sends a conflicting message and undermines the credibility of their advice on lifestyle interventions.

Picture this: a resident doctor enters the examination room, dispensing sage advice on the virtues of exercise, extolling its benefits for cardiovascular health, weight management, and stress reduction. Meanwhile, behind closed doors, the same doctor laments their own sedentary lifestyle, blaming long hours, hectic schedules, and the demanding nature of their profession for their lack of exercise.

Contrary to popular belief, the life of a doctor is not a continuous parade of brisk walks down hospital corridors, with the stethoscope swinging like a pendulum of physical activity. In reality, much of a doctor's day is spent in sedentary pursuits – hunched over desks, glued to computer screens, or seated in endless meetings. The only cardio workout may come from the occasional sprint to the operating room or the mad dash to catch up on rounds.

Despite their knowledge of nutrition and the importance of maintaining a healthy weight, many doctors find themselves succumbing to the temptations of comfort food and sedentary indulgence. The once svelte physiques of medical school give way to the soft contours of stress-eating and desk-bound inertia.

Stress, Sweat, and Self-Care: The Trifecta of Neglect

The culture within the medical community often glorifies sacrifice and self-neglect in the name of dedication to patient care. Doctors may feel guilty or selfish for taking time away from their work to prioritize their own health and well-being. This ingrained mindset, coupled with the pressure to excel in a highly competitive field, can make it challenging for doctors to carve out time for exercise.

The Wellness Paradox: Healing Others, Hurting Themselves

In their quest to heal others, doctors often neglect their own well-being, falling victim to the paradox of wellness. While they champion the importance of self-care and preventive health measures, they may neglect the very practices they preach. The healer becomes the patient, trapped in a cycle of neglect and self-sacrifice.

Residency marks the debut of our professional journey, a phase defined by exhaustive hours, erratic meal times, and reliance on junk food, often leading to declining physical health for most of us. Poor dietary choices and insufficient physical activity inevitably lead to physical deterioration, compromising our performance in our respective fields.

During my first month of residency, the unfamiliar environment led to a weight loss of 6 kgs as I struggled to find time for meals. Although I regained the lost weight later, the process likely involved muscle loss during weight loss and fat gain during the recovery phase. I consumed whatever was convenient on my way to work, with the main challenge being the inconsistency of meal times and varied stress coping mechanisms.

One of the primary culprits behind residents bad food habits is the relentless time crunch of medical practice. Long hours, irregular schedules, and the demanding nature of patient care leave little time for meal planning, grocery shopping, and home cooking. As a result, most residents often rely on fast food, vending machine snacks, and cafeteria fare to fuel their busy days, sacrificing nutritional quality for convenience. The very individuals tasked with promoting healthy eating may find themselves trapped in a cycle of convenience over conscious eating, prioritizing speed and accessibility over nutritional value. While samosas and coffee were the go-to food items during emergency duties for many, some turned to smoking cigarettes and consuming junk food to manage stress.

Stress Eating and Emotional Resilience: Coping Mechanisms in Crisis: In the high-pressure environment of medicine, stress eating often becomes a coping mechanism for doctors grappling with the demands of patient care, administrative burdens, and the specter of burnout. Comfort foods offer solace in times of stress, providing a temporary reprieve from the relentless pressure of medical practice. Many residents may turn to food as a source of emotional comfort and resilience in the face of adversity. The prevalence of unhealthy coping mechanisms can be attributed to a lack of understanding on how to effectively deal with stress, often seeking quick dopamine boosts. Is stress the sole factor? While not everyone in residency may agree, deep down, most of us wished for better coping strategies to navigate the demands of residency more effectively.

Ah, *"Chai and Sutta"* – the quintessential ritual in residency life. Nothing quite like bonding over tea and cigarettes, discussing the day's trials and tribulations with colleagues. Truly the highlight of the day for some souls.

"When you're mentally drained, engage in physical activity, conversely, when you're physically fatigued, stimulate your mind".

Throughout residency, I often found myself mentally fatigued, even after nights of good sleep. It wasn't until I realized that the lack of exercise was the underlying cause. Incorporating workouts into my routine not only refreshed my mind but also provided a dopamine boost, with improved physical fitness as a bonus. Most of you would naturally gravitate towards healthier eating habits once you start exercising—it becomes a catalyst for positive change. Exercise, in any form is the ultimate coping mechanism one could cultivate.

Exercise

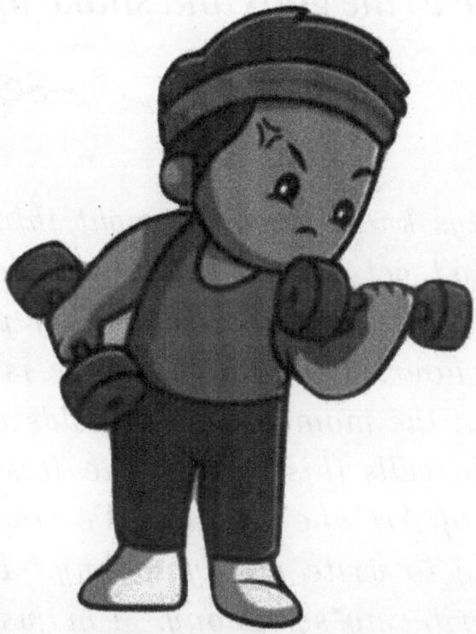

Strategies for Incorporating Fitness into Residency

1. Schedule regular exercise sessions: Despite busy schedules, we can prioritize fitness by scheduling regular exercise sessions into our daily routine. This may involve early morning workouts before the start of the workday, evening gym sessions after completing clinical duties, or even brief exercise breaks during shifts. I know it seems impossible to find time! I remember struggling to find time during my 1st residency but now during Urology residency I make time 3-4 times a week for some form of workout. Most of the times its late at 10-11 pm on my off calls. Retrospectively in MS, I could make time if I wanted, but I guess I gave reasons to myself. Here is what Greek philosopher Seneca had to say about lack of time:

"I don't complain about the lack of time.. what little I have will go far enough. Today—this day—will achieve what no tomorrow will fail to speak about. I will lay siege to the gods and shake up the world."

–Seneca, Medea

We almost always know what the right thing to do is. We know we shouldn't get upset, take things personally, order unhealthy food from Swiggy or Zomato, or procrastinate on focusing for an hour. The real challenge is choosing to do the right thing in the moment. What holds us back? Author Steven Pressfield calls this force "The Resistance." In his book 'The War of Art', he writes, "We don't tell ourselves, 'I'm never going to write my symphony.' Instead, we say, 'I'm going to write my symphony.' I'm just going to start tomorrow." Today, not tomorrow, is the day to begin making good choices.

2. Choose activities that fit your lifestyle: Finding time for exercise during residency can be challenging, so it's essential to choose activities that are convenient and enjoyable. This could include brisk walks during breaks, cycling to work, participating in group fitness classes, or following online workout videos that can be done at home or in the hospital gym. If you enjoy sports, playing your favorite sport can be an excellent and sustainable way to stay active. Personally, I enjoy watching UFC in my free time and have always been interested in learning boxing. Residency, however, didn't leave me with enough time to pursue it formally. So, I bought a punching bag and gloves, allowing me to fit in a good workout whenever I want, doing something I'm interested in learning.

3. Focus on High-Intensity Interval Training (HIIT): For people who are not into sports could find HIIT workouts more time appropriate. HIIT workouts are short, intense bursts of exercise followed by brief periods of rest or low-intensity activity. These workouts are time-efficient and can be completed in as little as 20-30 minutes, making them ideal for busy resident doctors looking to maximize their workout effectiveness in limited time. A short 20-30 mins workout while someone is guiding you online is probably easier to stick with.

4. Recovery and Rest: In addition to exercise, adequate rest and recovery are essential for maintaining physical health and preventing injury. You could ensure you get enough sleep each night, practice stress-reducing activities such as mindfulness or yoga, and listen to your body to avoid overtraining or burnout. If you were not very sporty growing up, remember stretching is as important as the workout.

Nutrition

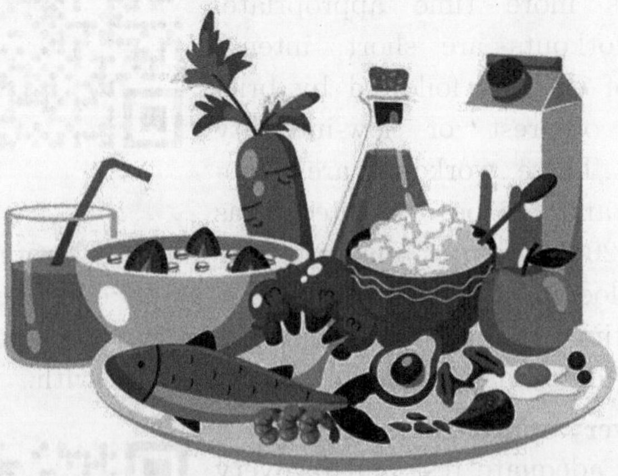

Food Habits for Residents

1. Nutrient intake and energy levels: Proper nutrition is essential for providing yourself with the energy and nutrients you need to sustain long shifts and demanding workloads. A balanced diet rich in whole foods, including fruits, vegetables, lean proteins, whole grains, and healthy fats, provides the necessary nutrients to fuel physical and cognitive performance. Nowadays, fast food is such a staple that if you opt for grilled kebabs or salads, people will look at you like you're on some extreme health kick. They'll probably ask, "Are you on a diet?" No, it's just called eating normal food, not embarking on a dietary pilgrimage!

2. Immune function and disease prevention: The demanding nature of residency, coupled with exposure to sick patients and irregular sleep patterns, can weaken the immune system and increase the risk of illness. A diet rich in vitamins, minerals, and antioxidants supports immune function, helping resident doctors stay healthy and resilient in the face of potential infections. We often find residents taking few months of sabitical due to TB, long absence due to dengue fever & innumerable episodes of URTI and gastroenteritis. During COVID-19, many suffered due to weak immune systems.

3. Mental health and mood regulation: Emerging research suggests a strong connection between diet and mental health, with certain nutrients playing a role in mood regulation and emotional well-being. Consuming a balanced diet that includes foods rich in omega-3 fatty acids, B vitamins, and magnesium may help support mental health and reduce the risk of mood disorders such as depression and anxiety.

4. Long-term health and disease prevention: Establishing healthy eating habits during residency sets the foundation for long-term health and wellness. By prioritizing nutritious foods and minimizing the consumption of processed foods, sugary beverages, and excessive amounts of caffeine, resident can reduce their risk of developing chronic diseases such as obesity, diabetes, and heart disease later in life. Keep an eye for HbA1C & Lipid profile during residency.

Strategies for Maintaining Healthy Food Habits during Residency

1. Meal Planning and Preparation

In India, meal planning often involves incorporating traditional dishes made from fresh, locally sourced ingredients. Resident can utilize their days time to batch cook nutritious meals such as *dal, sabzi,* and rice, which can be stored and reheated throughout the day. Packing homemade snacks like fruit chaat, sprouts, or homemade yogurt with nuts can provide energy during long shifts. The most preferable option is to have a tiffin service, at least for afternoon meals; as you could eat something wherever you could get some time. Protein bars can be good alternatives for a quick bite and are always handy in ones' back backs. I always had protein bars in my backpack during my 1st year. Currently my breakfast is something like a fruit and coffee or some muesli with milk. My afternoon meal is a tiffin service that provides me with 6 egg whites everyday in my lunch. Dinner is cooked by my cook. So this planning allows me to worry less about what to eat and I end up eating nutritious food.

2. Mindful Eating Practices

With the abundance of street food and tempting snacks available in India, it's important to practice mindful eating. This involves being aware of portion sizes, choosing healthier options like grilled kebabs or roasted peanuts over fried snacks, and savoring the flavors of traditional Indian cuisine, which is rich in spices and nutrients. Portion control is probably the most feasible option. You'll mostly eat what's available, but don't let your emotions drive you to eat as a coping mechanism. Many of us tend to eat when we're stressed, a habit formed in childhood when someone would cheer us up with food. This coping mechanism can become problematic. Practice portion control and consider using calorie-tracking apps. Using these apps even for just two weeks can make you more aware of your calorie and macronutrient intake. Understanding the basics of BMR and calorie counting will help you gain a better grasp of nutrition. Even gaining 1 kg every 2 months can add around 15-20 kgs by the end of your residency. If you're planning to lose weight, remember you gained the weight over a long period. Don't try to lose 10 kgs in 3 months when you gained it in 3 years. You'll probably regain it!

3. Stay Hydrated

In the Indian climate, staying hydrated is crucial, especially during hot and humid days. You could prioritize drinking plenty of water, coconut water, or *nimbu pani* to stay hydrated and replenish electrolytes. Avoiding excessive consumption of sugary chai or caffeinated beverages and opting for herbal teas or buttermilk can help maintain hydration levels without added sugar or caffeine.

4. Seek Out Healthy Food Options

Despite the allure of unhealthy options like samosas or pakoras in hospital cafeterias, healthier alternatives are often within reach. Exploring nearby restaurants or local eateries can uncover nutritious choices like *dal roti*, grilled chicken or fish, and fresh salads, aligning with your food preferences. Opting to have a cook prepare meals is an excellent choice, though it may be more practical if at least one person is available at home (As time of the cook's duty can vary).

5. Multivitamins and Supplements

Multivitamins and supplements can help fill potential nutritional gaps in the diet, ensuring you receive essential vitamins and minerals necessary for overall health and well-being. Immune Support with supplements such as vitamin C, vitamin D, and zinc, may help support immune function, reducing the risk of infections and illnesses, which is particularly important in the high-exposure environment of residency. I still remember the time when a friend of mine had stress # due to lack of vitamin D3 and calcium. While you may start multivitamins and supplements, remember it has potential for overdose. Taking excessive amounts of certain vitamins and minerals through supplementation can lead to toxicity and adverse effects. You should be cautious not to exceed recommended dosages. Not all supplements are rigorously regulated, and quality can vary between brands.

Addressing fitness and nutrition during residency is undoubtedly easier said than done. Despite understanding the importance of these practices, many residents including myself, have struggled to implement them consistently during the demanding training period. In my own experience, I encountered challenges during my General Surgery residency but I have since made significant improvements, particularly during my Urology Residency. It all comes down to setting priorities.

Prioritizing personal health can be difficult when faced with the relentless demands of patient care. There's a temptation to prioritize the well-being of others over our own, even if it means neglecting our own health in the process. However, it's essential to recognize that neglecting our health can have long-term consequences, potentially leading to conditions like hypertension, diabetes, or dyslipidemia. Starting medications to manage these conditions can serve as a wake-up call, reminding us of the importance of self-care and the need to prioritize our own health alongside that of our patients. It's a reminder that we cannot effectively care for others if we neglect our own well-being.

Ultimately, achieving balance during residency requires making conscious choices and establishing boundaries. It involves recognizing that self-care is not selfish but necessary for sustainable practice and long-term success in the medical field. By setting priorities and finding ways to incorporate fitness and nutrition into our daily lives, we can better care for ourselves and, in turn, provide better care for our patients. If a group of friends do these activities together, it can be more effective. Going for workout sessions with friends can be a great way to relax and stay fit. Encouraging each other to eat healthy helps everyone stick to a healthier diet.

Healthy Hustle

In residency's wild, frantic race,
We try to find a balanced space.
Boundaries drawn with hopeful might,
So we don't turn into zombies overnight.

Self-care's not selfish, let's be clear,
It's just our way to persevere.
Setting priorities, a survival knack,
In fitness and food, we get on track.

With friends, this all becomes a game,
We dodge the stress, avoid the shame.
Workout sessions, a sweaty jest,
Together, we strive to do our best.

"Eat healthy!" we cheer with glee,
As we all eye the salad reluctantly.
But together, we stand, a mighty crew,
In this madness, we push through.

So here's to balance, with a wink and grin,
In residency's chaos, we find our spin.
Sustainable practice and a healthy diet,
In this circus, we find our might!

Dr. Alhad Naragude

Chapter 8

FINANCES

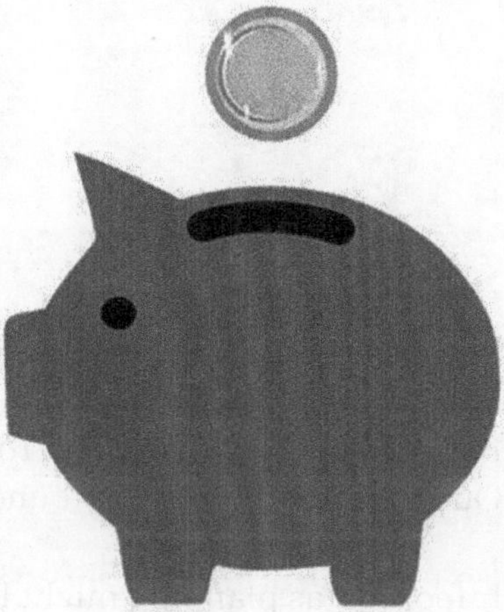

For many of us, residency represents our inaugural professional experience. We serve in hospitals and receive compensation for our work, which may be the first substantial income we've managed independently. The extent of our financial acumen varies, often influenced by our familial backgrounds. Additionally, as employees, we are subject to taxes, further complicating our financial landscape. Amidst the demands of residency, which can be overwhelming on their own, the foresight to make sound financial decisions for the future may be lacking. Balancing new financial responsibilities with the rigors of training adds an extra layer of complexity, making it challenging to prioritize long-term financial planning.

Furthermore, the transition into residency typically coincides with a period of significant life changes. Many residents relocate to new cities or even countries, requiring adjustments to living expenses and financial priorities. Amidst this upheaval, the importance of financial planning for the future may not receive the attention it deserves.

Stethoscopes to Savings

In the race of residency, foresight's thin,
Financial planning? Where to begin?
Balancing bills with endless rounds,
Our fiscal logic often confounds.

Important as planning might be,
It's overshadowed by the latest IV.
Personal pursuits and money talk,
Lost in the shuffle of the hospital walk.

Med school's wisdom on healing's profound,
But budgeting tips? Nowhere to be found.
We master the scalpel, the needle's grace,
But managing cash? We're all over the
place.

With schedules packed tight, free time's
rare,
Financial books? We wouldn't dare.
Default behaviors, reacting in haste,
Our bank accounts? What a waste!

Stethoscopes to Savings

No formal training on taxes or debt,
We diagnose well, but our budgets are never set.
Yet there's hope in sight, with resources to find,
Books, online courses, to ease our mind.

Let's foster a chat about money woes,
Share tips and tricks, see how it goes.
Building portfolios while cracking a joke,
We'll navigate finance, and not make ourselves broke!

So here's to the residents in financial strife,
Balancing budgets with medical life.
With efforts and help, we'll sort out our stash,
And maybe, just maybe, not end up cash-crash!

Dr. Alhad Naragude

Moreover, the demanding nature of residency leaves little time for personal pursuits, let alone comprehensive financial education. Residents often find themselves consumed by clinical duties, leaving little mental bandwidth to delve into complex financial matters. As a result, they may rely on default financial behaviors or simply react to immediate needs without considering long-term implications.

The lack of formal financial education in medical training programs exacerbates the challenge. While medical schools prepare residents to excel in clinical practice, they often neglect to provide adequate guidance on financial literacy and management. As a result, many residents enter the workforce with limited knowledge of budgeting, investing, debt management, and tax planning.

During my time as an intern, I witnessed a common practice among some resident doctors who would entrust their ATM cards to interns, encouraging them to freely spend as they pleased on a routine basis. The potential consequences of frivolous spending, driven by a lack of financial management skills, could eventually lead to substantial regrets in the future.

I'm stuck between "I need to save money" and "You only live once."

By proactively seeking out resources, such as books, online courses, or financial advisors, residents can gain the knowledge and skills needed to make informed financial decisions. Moreover, fostering a culture of open communication and support within residency programs can facilitate discussions about financial challenges and strategies for navigating them effectively.

"Financial freedom is available to those who learn about it and work for it."

–Robert Kiyosaki

Challenges Faced

1. Stipends: The stipends provided to medical residents in India often fall short of covering their living expenses, particularly in major cities with high costs of living. This financial strain often leads to stress and anxiety among residents. Stipends typically range from 40,000 to approximately 110,000 rupees per month. For instance, if monthly expenditures amount to around 30,000 rupees, the potential savings can vary significantly based on the stipend received. Depending on the stipend, residents could save anywhere from 10,000 to 80,000 rupees per month. Over a three-year residency period, this translates to cumulative savings ranging from 360,000 to 2,880,000 rupees. Hence, it's crucial to consider the stipend amount when selecting an institution for residency training. At times depending on the city of your choice the basic rent you pay to live with your family (if married) or friends might be upwards of 40,000 for a mere 1 BHK!

2. Loans: Medical education in India can be expensive in private setups and some residents graduate with significant student loan debt. Balancing loan repayments with living expenses on a limited income can pose a significant challenge, impacting financial stability and long-term planning. Not just student loans, there could be home, car loans and other miscellaneous EMIs' that one could be paying to support their family needs.

3. Long working hours: Medical residency is notorious for its long working hours and unpredictable schedules. Residents often have little time or energy to devote to managing their finances effectively.

4. Limited opportunities for additional income: The demanding nature of residency often leaves little time for any freelance or partime jobs. Balancing work and additional income-generating activities can be challenging and may contribute to burnout.

Strategies for Financial Management

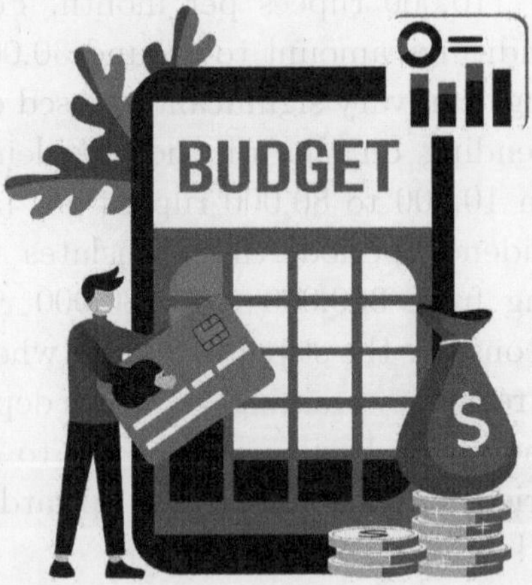

1. Budgeting: Budgeting is a fundamental aspect of financial management, enabling to meticulously monitor their expenditures and prioritize critical necessities. It entails allocating funds strategically for key expenses such as rent, utilities, groceries, transportation, loan repayments, and savings, thereby ensuring that expenditures remain within the confines of their income.

For instance, setting aside a predetermined portion of income for rent ensures that housing expenses are covered without straining financial resources. Similarly, allocating funds for utilities guarantees the continuous provision of essential services while avoiding any unexpected disruptions due to non-payment. Additionally, earmarking a specific amount for groceries facilitates responsible spending on food essentials, promoting both financial stability and healthy nutrition.

"It's not your salary that makes you rich, it's your spending habits."

2. Building an emergency fund: Creating an emergency fund is imperative for medical residents to safeguard against unforeseen expenses or financial crises. Every month strive to allocate a portion of your stipend or salary into a designated savings account until you've amassed enough to cover 3 to 6 months' worth of living expenses.

3. Managing loans: If you have student loans, explore options for repayment plans, loan consolidation, or refinancing to manage monthly payments effectively. If you have other loans like car loan, home loan, etc. manage the debt EMI as per your stipend. Repaying education loans on time helps you establish a positive credit history, which is advantageous for future financial pursuits, like securing a mortgage or starting a clinic/hospital. Additionally, it fosters financial discipline and responsibility, laying a solid foundation for sound financial management in the future.

4. Prioritizing health insurance: Ensure that you have adequate health insurance coverage to protect yourself from unexpected medical expenses. Though medical expenses in India are cheaper compared to developed nations, it can hurt your savings.

5. Developing financial literacy: Take the time to educate yourself about personal finance management through books, online resources, or financial planning workshops. Understanding concepts such as budgeting, investing, debt management, and insurance can empower you to make informed financial decisions throughout your residency and beyond. Learning to use credit cards to improve your credit score. Learning what credit score means and how exactly does it affect your ability to take financial leverage with loans. Even if you're not a fan of math or accounting, it's important to recognize their real-life significance. Sure, you might have a parent, sibling, or friend who's a CA handling your taxes and managing your savings in PPFs or FDs, but you should understand what all that entails! For example, most of my taxes are still done by my father's CA. During my MS, I never invested money on my own; I'd simply hand over a major portion of my savings to my father to manage and invest. He took care of everything.

The importance of financial literacy hit me when I considered my educational path. With such an extended education, I realized I wouldn't start earning a substantial income until 8-10 years after my friends in other fields. While learning communication and professional skills in residency might make you a competent doctor; understanding finances? That's something you'll likely need to learn on your own.

6. Investing wisely: Start investing early, even with small amounts with investment options such as mutual funds, SIPs', Equity, Fixed Deposits, etc as per your risk appetite Consult with a financial advisor to develop an investment strategy that aligns with your financial goals and risk tolerance. Compound interest is a powerful concept in investing that allows you to grow your wealth exponentially over time. Initially, the growth may seem gradual, but as time passes, the rate of growth accelerates, resulting in a larger and larger investment base leading to a snowball effect & can turn even modest investments into substantial sums over extended periods.

In India, many from our parents' generation have tales of someone who lost all their money in the stock market. These cautionary stories have led to widespread reluctance to invest in equities. Rarely does anyone dig into the specifics of what actually caused those losses. The pervasive fear has kept us from understanding the details, dampening our interest in exploring the stock market.

On the flip side, there's a growing crowd enamored with the idea of hitting the financial jackpot, expecting the stock market to turn their modest investments into a 5-10x windfall within a year. Stories of rags-to-riches, like those Bitcoin billionaires who are now sipping cocktails on their private islands, are all over the internet. However, expecting such returns is like betting on a lottery ticket: it's more about luck than savvy investing. Unless someone's consistently pulling those numbers, it's not skill, it's just a very lucky rabbit's foot at play.

This fear and fascination create a fascinating dichotomy: one generation playing it safer than a bubble-wrapped egg, and another dreaming of becoming overnight tycoons. What we often overlook is the power of education and due diligence in investments. By understanding market fundamentals, risks, and the beauty of long-term growth, you can bridge the gap between fear and speculation. Investing isn't about striking gold overnight; it's more about making smart, informed decisions and having the patience of a saint.

1. *Stocks:* Stocks represent ownership stakes in publicly traded companies. Investors purchase shares of stock, entitling them to a portion of the company's profits and voting rights in corporate decisions. Stocks offer the potential for significant returns over the long term but are also subject to market volatility and fluctuations. They are ideal for investors with a *higher risk tolerance* seeking capital appreciation. There are numerous investment options, such as equity shares and futures & options, that can yield double-digit returns. However, these come with considerable risks, so it's advisable to first understand the basics of the market and learn how to analyze a company's financial statements. Start small if you're interested and once you have some hold on basics, you could invest further. Advantage of stock market if that your money is liquid. You can comfortably sell your shares and exit your positions. This gives you handy money as per your needs and you can stay invested at the same time.

2. *Bonds:* Bonds are debt securities issued by governments, municipalities, or corporations to raise capital. When an investor purchases a bond, they are essentially lending money to the issuer in exchange for periodic interest payments and the return of the principal amount at maturity. Bonds are generally considered safer than stocks but offer lower potential returns. They are suitable for *conservative investors* seeking steady income and capital preservation.

3. *Mutual Funds:* Mutual funds pool money from multiple investors to invest in a diversified portfolio of stocks, bonds, or other securities. They are professionally managed and offer investors instant diversification and access to a wide range of assets. Mutual funds come in various types, including equity funds, bond funds, and hybrid funds, catering to different risk preferences and investment objectives. They are suitable for investors seeking diversification and professional management. Currently Indian MFs' have SIPs' of over

20,000 crores every month. There are high risk funds giving returns of over 40% CAGR over the last 3 years!

4. *Exchange-Traded Funds (ETFs):* ETFs are similar to mutual funds but trade on stock exchanges like individual stocks. They offer the same benefits of diversification and professional management but with greater flexibility and liquidity. ETFs track various indices, sectors, or asset classes and are available in a wide range of options, allowing investors to customize their portfolios according to specific investment strategies. They are suitable for investors seeking low-cost, tax-efficient investment vehicles with intraday trading capabilities.

5. *Real Estate Investment Trusts (REITs):* REITs are companies that own, operate, or finance income-generating real estate properties. Investors can buy shares of REITs, which provide exposure to the real estate market without the need to directly purchase properties. REITs typically generate income through rental properties, and they are required to distribute a significant portion of their taxable income to shareholders in the form of dividends. REITs offer diversification, income, and potential capital appreciation, making them suitable for investors seeking exposure to real estate with liquidity and transparency.

Here is a link to an online Masterclass by Mr. Sharan Hegde that could act as a starting point for your financial planning. I saw one of my juniors using it to have a basic understanding of personal finances.

(***Disclaimer:*** I'm not sponsored or afflicted with the course or the program).